AF687091

Intensive Short-Term Dynamic Psychotherapy for Beginners

A Clear, Practical Introduction to ISTDP: Core Concepts, the Triangle of Conflict, and Working with Emotion and Defense

Valentine George Lucas

Copyright 2026 by Valentine George Lucas. All rights reserved. No part of this book may be reproduced, stored in a retrieval system, or transmitted in any form or by any means, electronic, mechanical, photocopying, recording, or otherwise, without the prior written permission of the publisher, except for brief quotations used in reviews.

Disclaimer

This book is for educational purposes only. It is an introduction to a professional psychotherapy model, not a training in that model, and reading it does not qualify anyone to practice Intensive Short-Term Dynamic Psychotherapy. The techniques described here require formal training, supervision, and a professional license to use with clients. Nothing in this book is medical advice, psychological treatment, or a substitute for care from a qualified professional.

All names, characters, organizations, and scenarios described in the stories and examples in this book are fictional composites created for teaching purposes. Any resemblance to real individuals, living or dead, or to actual organizations or events is coincidental.

The author and publisher make no warranties, express or implied, about the completeness, accuracy, or fitness of this material for any particular purpose, and shall not be liable for any loss, injury, or damage allegedly arising from the use of the information contained in this book. Readers assume full responsibility for the use of this material. If you are struggling with your mental health, please reach out to a licensed professional in your area.

Published in 2026

ISBN 979-8-90599-687-0

Table of Contents

Preface

Over the past three decades, outcome research in psychotherapy has quietly rewritten what the field believes about how fast deep change can happen. Among the approaches driving that revision, few have generated more interest, or more rumor, than Intensive Short-Term Dynamic Psychotherapy. Born from Habib Davanloo's filmed sessions in Montreal and mapped for teaching by the British researcher David Malan, ISTDP now supports international training networks and a growing meta-analytic evidence base, while the number of accredited trainers remains small enough that provision is thin in most of the world. Interest in the model has plainly outgrown the teaching materials available to newcomers.

ISTDP is a psychodynamic therapy built on a specific claim: that the avoidance of emotion, learned early in important relationships, drives most of the symptoms that bring people to treatment, and that the direct bodily experience of avoided feeling, in the presence of an active and allied therapist, produces deep and lasting change. It differs from classical psychoanalysis in its pace and activity, from cognitive approaches in its target, and its central diagram, the triangle of conflict, is frequently confused online with the unrelated Karpman drama triangle. Precision about these distinctions matters, and this book supplies it from the first chapter.

The problem facing the curious reader is structural. The model's literature is written almost entirely for clinicians already inside it: advanced technique manuals, dense theoretical volumes, and introductory texts priced as academic hardbacks. Reliable information about training routes, costs, and entry requirements is scattered across provider websites. Into that vacuum has flowed a caricature, the confrontational therapy of the old videotapes, which misrepresents a field that has spent forty years refining calibration, anxiety regulation, and alliance.

This book is a plain-language introduction to the whole model. It teaches the triangle of conflict and the triangle of persons, the three bodily pathways of anxiety, the compassionate logic of working with defenses, the structure of a first session, the meaning of therapeutic pressure inside an explicit alliance, the graded adaptation for fragile clients, and the honest state of the evidence. Every concept arrives through realistic stories and worked examples before theory, and every chapter addresses what to do when the ideas fail to land. The intended outcome is practical: a reader who can follow the model's clinical reasoning, evaluate its fit, and, if they choose, approach formal training with a mapped path, known costs, and a structured ninety-day self-study plan.

The book stands on its own and requires no companion volume, though its closing chapter recommends a reading order for those continuing deeper into the clinical literature. It is written first for practicing therapists and counselors who are weighing this model, and it will serve students of psychology and psychotherapy, clinicians trained in adjacent approaches, and general readers with a serious interest in how emotional change works.

What this book cannot do is equally clear. It is not a training, it confers no license to use the techniques it describes, and it promises no clinical or personal result; the interventions discussed here belong in the hands of professionals working under supervision, and the text marks that boundary wherever it applies. Its purpose is to open a door that has stayed closed too long: a clear, honest, affordable understanding of ISTDP for the reader standing at the beginning.

Introduction

Morag heard about it the way most therapists do. Sideways.

She was 41, a counselor with eight years of practice behind her, solid CBT training, and a caseload she mostly felt good about. Then her consultation group watched a video. A therapist somewhere in Canada sat across from a man who had been in and out of treatment for a decade. Within twenty minutes, the man was sobbing about his father in a way that felt less like a breakdown and more like a dam finally doing what dams are eventually supposed to do. The therapist had not pushed him into it, exactly. She had just refused, gently and relentlessly, to let him slide away from himself.

Someone in the group said, "That is ISTDP."

Morag went home and searched the term. She found four letters that stood for Intensive Short-Term Dynamic Psychotherapy, a founder named Davanloo, a concept called the triangle of conflict, and a stack of books that all seemed to be written for people who already understood them. One was subtitled Advanced Psychotherapy Techniques. Another had Mastering in the title. A workshop near her cost more than her car insurance. She closed twelve tabs and felt the specific discouragement of someone standing outside a party listening to everyone laugh.

If any part of that is familiar, this book was written for you.

Here is what this book will do. It will explain ISTDP in plain English, from the ground up, assuming no psychoanalytic background at all. It will teach you the model's two famous triangles until you can see them operating in real clinical material. It will show you how ISTDP therapists read anxiety in the body and meet defenses without shaming anyone. It will walk you through a first session, a breakthrough, and the quieter work that follows. It will answer the question you are too polite to ask out loud, which is what all this costs and how you would actually train. And it will be honest about the model's controversies instead of pretending they do not exist.

Here is what this book will not do. It will not make you an ISTDP therapist. Reading about pressure and challenge does not license you to use them, any more than reading about surgery licenses you to operate. Throughout the book you will find clear markers of what you can safely begin noticing and practicing now, and what belongs only in formal training with supervision. Those markers are not legal boilerplate. They are the same boundaries good ISTDP trainers hold, and holding them is part of understanding the model.

One more thing before you start. You might be thinking that everyone else in your field already understands this and you are late. You are not. Most therapists know ISTDP only as a rumor, the intense one, the one with the videos. The gap between hearing about this model and understanding it is enormous, and almost nobody has crossed it. You are about to.

Before Chapter 1.0, do one small thing. Write down the name of one client who talks about feelings without ever seeming to feel them, and one question you hope this model can answer. Keep the note somewhere you will find it. We will come back to both.

Chapter 1.0: What ISTDP Actually Is

Lorcan almost skipped the seminar. He was a therapist in his late fifties, thirty years into a career, and he had seen enough new models arrive with trumpets and leave without them. But the presenter played a video, and Lorcan leaned forward despite himself.

On the screen, a woman was explaining her marriage in the flat, careful voice of someone reading a weather report about their own house burning down. The therapist said, "You are describing something painful, but I notice your voice stays even. What do you feel right now, as you tell me this?" The woman paused. Her hands tightened. "I suppose I should feel upset." The therapist did not move on. "That is what you think you should feel. What do you actually feel, here, in your body, this moment?" A long silence. Then the woman's face did something complicated, and she said, quietly, "Angry. I think I have been angry for six years."

Six years. Lorcan thought about his own caseload, the clients who supposed they should feel things, and how often he had accepted the weather report and moved on. Whatever this model was, it had just done in four minutes what he sometimes failed to do in four months.

This chapter gives you the plain-English answer to the question Lorcan asked the presenter afterward: what is this, actually? By the end, you will be able to define ISTDP in two sentences, explain what each word in its long name means, describe how a session differs from most therapy you have seen, and give an honest one-paragraph account of the evidence behind it. That is the foundation everything else in this book builds on.

1.1 The Two Sentence Answer

Here is ISTDP in two sentences. It is a therapy built on the idea that emotional avoidance causes most of the suffering that brings people to treatment, and that helping people directly experience the feelings they have spent a lifetime avoiding produces deep and lasting change. It is called intensive because it goes after that avoided feeling actively rather than waiting for it, short-term because working this way compresses change into months rather than years, and dynamic because it works with the parts of emotional life that operate outside awareness (Coughlin Della Selva, 2004).

Read those sentences again, because they contain a quiet radical claim. Most therapies treat symptoms. Depression, panic, chronic self-criticism, the stomach that knots before every meeting. ISTDP treats those things as the visible exhaust of an invisible engine. The engine is a person's system for not feeling what they feel. Somewhere early in life, usually inside important relationships, certain feelings became dangerous to have. Anger toward a parent you depended on. Grief nobody would sit with. Love that got punished. The child's solution was brilliant and costly: bury the feeling, and build machinery to keep it buried. Decades later, the machinery is still running, and the maintenance costs have become symptoms (Frederickson, 2013).

An ISTDP therapist, then, is not primarily asking what is wrong with you. They are asking what you are avoiding, how you avoid it, and what it costs you. And rather than only talking about that avoidance, they invite you to stop doing it, right there in the room, while someone steady sits with you. The feeling you finally have, instead of the feeling you have been managing, is where the healing happens.

1.2 Unpacking the Long Name

Every word in Intensive Short-Term Dynamic Psychotherapy is doing a job, so let's take them one at a time.

Intensive describes the stance, not the volume. The therapist is active. They ask specific questions, notice avoidance the moment it appears, and keep inviting the client back to their inner experience. The aim, as the founder framed it, is to help the person experience their warded-off feelings as fully as possible rather than in safe, partial doses (Davanloo, 1990). If most therapy is a slow walk alongside the client, ISTDP is closer to a focused expedition with a clear destination.

Short-term is a result, not a gimmick. Nobody is watching a stopwatch. But when a therapy targets the engine of symptoms rather than the exhaust, change tends to arrive faster. The classic texts describe substantial character-level change in a few dozen sessions for many clients, which was a scandalous claim when psychoanalysis expected years (Coughlin Della Selva, 2004). Treatment length still varies with the person. Some finish in ten sessions. Fragile clients, whom you will meet in Chapter 9.0, need longer, gentler versions.

Dynamic means the model takes the unconscious seriously. Not as a spooky basement, but as a plain observable fact: people ward off feelings without knowing they are doing it, and those feelings press for expression anyway, showing up as anxiety, symptoms, and repeating relationship patterns. Dynamic also means the model expects your old relationships to walk into the therapy room with you, a phenomenon called **transference**, which simply means treating a present person with feelings that belong to a past one. Chapter 4.0 covers this properly.

Psychotherapy you already know. Two people, one room or one screen, and the strange reliable magic of honest attention.

1.3 Example

Consider a scenario like this one. Keva was 38, an operations manager, and her doctor was tired of finding nothing. Headaches four days a week, scans clean, blood work fine. The referral note said stress. Keva arrived at therapy with a bright, pleasant smile and said she really could not complain.

For three sessions with her previous therapist, she had reviewed her week, agreed that self-care was important, and kept the smile on. The headaches continued. Her new therapist worked dynamically. In the first session, she asked Keva for one specific recent moment the headache had spiked. Keva mentioned Sunday dinner, when her brother announced he was borrowing money from their mother. Again. As Keva described it, her jaw set and her voice stayed sweet.

The therapist said, "I notice you are smiling as you tell me this. What is the feeling underneath the smile, toward your brother?" Keva said she was not really a person who got angry. The therapist did not argue. She asked what Keva noticed in her body right now. "My head," Keva said slowly, "is starting to hurt."

That was the moment. Not a breakthrough, not tears, just a live demonstration: feeling stirred, the smile clamped down, and the pressure went somewhere. Over the following weeks, as Keva began letting the anger arrive as anger, something unglamorous happened. The headaches did not vanish, but they dropped to one a week, and Keva could predict them. Her relationship with her brother remained genuinely difficult. Some things a therapy cannot fix.

What this means for you: symptoms often sit exactly where avoided feeling goes. ISTDP is a systematic way of following the symptom back to the feeling. You do not need training to start noticing that trail in your own practice.

1.4 What a Session Looks Like

You might be thinking that this sounds reasonable in theory and wondering what it looks like at the level of actual minutes. Fair. Here is the texture.

An ISTDP session is specific. The therapist asks for concrete examples rather than summaries. Not how was your week, but tell me one moment this week the problem showed up, and walk me through it. Generalities are where feelings go to hide.

It is collaborative in an unusual way. Early on, the therapist and client build agreement about what they are there to do: to face, together, the feelings the client has been facing alone or not at all. ISTDP writers call the client's healthy wish to get well and be known the bedrock of the work, and the therapist appeals to it constantly (Frederickson, 2013).

It is attentive to the body. While the client talks, the therapist watches. Sighs, clenched hands, a fog rolling in behind the eyes. These are readouts of rising feeling and anxiety, and Chapter 5.0 will teach you the grammar of them.

And it is honest about avoidance. When the client changes the subject, goes vague, laughs the pain away, or explains instead of feeling, the therapist names it, kindly and without exception. Not as an accusation, but as an observation offered to an ally: do you notice we just moved away from your father the moment tears came?

If that sounds different from the therapy you were trained in, you are reading it correctly. It is also, for many clients, a relief. Someone finally declined to be fooled.

1.5 Example

Meet Orson. He was 52, a university lecturer, and he arrived at therapy with what he called low-grade lifelong depression and a truly impressive vocabulary for describing it. He had read more psychology than most therapists. He could discuss his childhood attachment patterns fluently, in the third person, the way a tour guide discusses a castle.

His previous therapies had been pleasant and useless, and he said so with a dry little laugh. His new therapist noticed the laugh. In the second session, Orson was narrating his mother's coldness with his usual polish, and the therapist said, "You describe this brilliantly. And I notice that while you describe it, nothing seems to happen in you. What do you feel toward her, right now, as you remember standing at that door?"

Orson began another explanation. The therapist gently interrupted. "That is your mind explaining her. I am asking what you feel toward her." There was a silence Orson later described as vertical. What came was not rage but grief, sudden and physical, and underneath it a wave of longing for his mother that embarrassed him more than any anger could have.

Orson did not become a different man in a month. His progress was slow and lurching, with two stretches where he seriously considered quitting because feeling worse than his baseline numbness frightened him. But by the end of the year, colleagues had noticed he laughed differently. His own words: the castle tour finally went inside.

What this means for you: intelligence and insight can be the most elegant avoidance system ever built. Watch for the clients who understand everything and feel nothing. They are often the ones this model was made for.

1.6 The Evidence in One Page

You will want to justify your interest, to your supervisor and to yourself, so here is the honest evidence summary.

ISTDP belongs to the family of short-term psychodynamic therapies, which have solid support overall. A Cochrane review of short-term psychodynamic psychotherapies for common mental disorders found significant benefits in the short and medium term for general, depressive, and anxiety symptoms, with effect sizes that grew at longer follow-up though several no longer reached statistical significance; the reviewers themselves urge caution, given limited data and heterogeneity between studies (Abbass et al., 2014). Psychodynamic therapy more broadly shows effect sizes comparable to other evidence-based treatments, with a pattern of continued improvement after therapy ends (Shedler, 2010). That synthesis drew immediate methodological objections in the same journal, chiefly that it pooled studies of very different diagnoses and quality, and the exchange is worth reading alongside it (Anestis et al., 2011).

For ISTDP specifically, a systematic review and meta-analysis of outcome research found meaningful improvements across a range of conditions, including treatment-resistant ones (Abbass, Town, & Driessen, 2012). A meta-analysis of experiential dynamic therapies, the wider family ISTDP anchors, reached similar conclusions (Lilliengren et al., 2016), and its ten-year update, covering fifty-seven randomized trials and more than four thousand patients, held to the same finding while widening the evidence to children, adolescents, and non-Western settings (Lilliengren et al., 2025). Effectiveness research in a real-world tertiary service found that clients improved and that in-session emotional breakthroughs were associated with better outcomes (Johansson, Town, & Abbass, 2014).

The honest caveats: many studies are small, some come from research groups invested in the model, and ISTDP has fewer large independent trials than CBT, which has a forty-year head start and an army of researchers. The fair summary is promising and growing, not proven beyond argument. Anyone who tells you otherwise, in either direction, is selling something.

1.7 When It Doesn't Work

The most common way this chapter fails is quietly, about a week from now, when you try to explain ISTDP to a colleague and hear yourself say it is the confrontational one where they make you feel your feelings. The definition collapses back into the rumor.

This is not a memory problem. It is a compression problem. You received a lot of new structure at once, and under pressure, the mind reaches for the cartoon version.

Three things to try. First, rehearse the two-sentence answer from section 1.1 out loud, twice, today. Saying it is different from reading it. Second, attach the definition to a person: retell Keva's story to yourself, because stories survive compression better than definitions. Third, notice one client this week who reports feelings without experiencing them, and silently label what you saw. One observation will anchor the concept better than three rereadings.

And if the definition still will not stick, let it go for now. The next four chapters each rebuild it from a different side. By Chapter 5.0 you will not be able to forget it if you try.

1.8 The Quick Version

ISTDP is a therapy built on one central claim: emotional avoidance is the engine of most psychological symptoms, and directly experiencing avoided feeling, in the presence of a steady ally, is the cure. Intensive describes the therapist's active stance. Short-term describes the compressed timeline that results. Dynamic means the model works with feelings and patterns that operate outside awareness, including the old relationships that walk into the room disguised as the new one.

Sessions are specific, body-aware, and honest about avoidance the moment it appears. The evidence base is genuinely encouraging, with meta-analytic support for ISTDP and its family of therapies, and it is still smaller than CBT's, which is worth saying plainly.

Most of all, hold on to the reframe. The question shifts from what is wrong with this person to what are they avoiding, how, and at what cost. If you take nothing else from this chapter, take the question. It will change what you notice by Friday.

Chapter 2.0: Where ISTDP Came From

Meeka's core training group met in a rented seminar room that smelled faintly of old coffee, and on the first morning, the trainer did something odd. Instead of starting with theory, she played a grainy video from the 1970s. The colors had faded to orange and teal. A psychiatrist with a heavy accent was interviewing a man about his failed marriages, and the psychiatrist would not let a single vague answer pass. Every time the man drifted, the psychiatrist brought him back, politely, insistently, like someone repeatedly returning a dropped wallet.

Meeka found it uncomfortable. Then, around minute forty, the man on the tape stopped fencing. His face changed. Decades of grief about his brother's death came through him in a way that made the whole seminar room go still, fifty years and a video transfer later.

The trainer paused the tape. "Everything we will study for three years," she said, "started because one stubborn man refused to believe this had to take a decade, and filmed everything to find out why it did not have to."

That stubborn man was Habib Davanloo, and this chapter tells the story of where ISTDP came from. You will get the problem Davanloo set out to solve, the unusual method he used to solve it, the British researcher whose maps became the model's teaching language, and the family tree of therapies that grew from this root. History may sound optional. It is not, because the field's culture, including its obsession with video, only makes sense once you know the origin story.

2.1 The Problem With the Couch

Start with the world Davanloo trained in. Mid-twentieth-century psychoanalysis was the prestige treatment of its day, and it had a dirty open secret: it was extraordinarily long, and its results were extraordinarily uneven. Analyses ran five days a week for years. Some patients transformed. Many circled. The method's own logic explained away its failures, because if you did not improve, you were resisting, and if you were resisting, you clearly needed more analysis.

Davanloo, a psychiatrist working in Montreal, found this unacceptable in a way that seems to have been temperamental as much as intellectual. He believed the healing core of psychoanalysis, the direct experience of previously unconscious feeling, was real. He also believed the delivery system was broken, protecting itself with unfalsifiable explanations and unlimited timelines (Davanloo, 1990).

He was not entirely alone. Earlier analysts had experimented with shorter, more active treatments, and a research tradition of brief dynamic therapy already existed at London's Tavistock Clinic, where David Malan was running some of the first serious outcome studies of short psychodynamic work (Malan, 1979). But nobody had cracked the central problem: how do you get past a lifetime of defenses quickly, without either bulldozing the patient or waiting years for the walls to lower on their own?

Hold that question, because everything in this book is a piece of Davanloo's answer to it.

2.2 The Camera Changes Everything

Davanloo's move sounds obvious now and was radical then: he pointed a camera at his sessions and watched the tapes. Not casually. Frame by frame, hour after hour, comparing what he did with what happened next, discarding interventions that produced compliance or stalemate and keeping the ones that produced genuine feeling (Davanloo, 1990).

Sit with how unusual this was. Therapy in that era was a black box. What happened in the room was reconstructed from the therapist's notes and memory, both famously flattering. Davanloo submitted himself to the tape, which flatters nobody. The tape showed him when his patients complied without changing. It showed him the exact moment a sigh appeared, a hand clenched, a patient went foggy. Over thousands of hours, patterns emerged that no one had described with such precision before: how feeling rises, how anxiety discharges through the body in distinct channels, how defenses mobilize in real time, and what a therapist can do at each juncture (Coughlin Della Selva, 2004).

Out of this came the method's spine. The therapist maintains steady pressure toward feeling. Resistance rises, and with it a strange energy Davanloo called complex transference feelings, the mixture of old rage, guilt, love, and grief now aimed at the therapist who will not go away. Handled correctly, the patient's own healthy side turns against the defenses, and the buried feeling breaks through, often bringing with it memories the person did not know they had (Davanloo, 1990). Handled incorrectly, you get a very unhappy patient, which is why Chapters 5.0, 8.0, and 9.0 exist.

This is also why ISTDP training still revolves around video today. The field was born from tape, and it trusts tape more than testimony. When you eventually train, your own sessions will go under that same honest light. Chapter 12.0 will help you make peace with that in advance.

2.3 Example

Take a person in this situation. Auli was a trainee clinical psychologist assigned to write a seminar paper on the history of brief therapy, and she resented it. History felt like homework while her classmates learned actual skills. She grabbed the oldest source on the reading list, Malan's outcome research, planning to skim.

She did not skim. What caught her was Malan's honesty about failure. Here was a researcher inside the psychoanalytic establishment publishing evidence that carefully selected patients could change deeply in twenty or thirty sessions, and that some long analyses achieved less than some short ones (Malan, 1979). The data was rough by modern standards. The willingness to look was not.

Then Auli hit the part of the story where Malan, in 1974, watched Davanloo's videotapes and became something close to an evangelist, beginning a collaboration that ran for more than a decade and lending his own teaching diagrams to the task of making Davanloo's dense clinical discoveries comprehensible (Malan, 1980). Auli had assumed the triangle diagrams in her handouts were generic therapy clip art. They were Malan's, drawn from older analytic sources and simplified by him years before he ever saw a Davanloo tape.

Her seminar paper came in two days late anyway, because Auli was a chronic deadline optimist and no amount of inspiration fixed that. But she stopped resenting the history. She had found the thing beginners rarely expect to find there: evidence that the field's founders were beginners too, watching tape, getting it wrong, and keeping only what worked.

What this means for you: the maps you are about to learn in Chapters 3.0 and 4.0 were forged from filmed evidence and outcome data, not armchair theory. You can lean your weight on them.

2.4 Malan and the Maps

David Malan deserves his own section, because his contribution is the language this book will teach you.

Malan was a British psychiatrist and researcher who spent his career at the Tavistock Clinic asking an unfashionable question: does this actually work, and for whom? His studies of brief psychodynamic therapy were among the first to link specific therapist behaviors, especially interpretations connecting present patterns to past relationships, with measured outcomes (Malan, 1979).

His most durable gift was a pair of diagrams, which he did not invent but did make usable. Malan was explicit about his debts. He took the three-person map from Karl Menninger, who had called it the triangle of insight, and he simplified the internal map out of the three-part interpretations his Tavistock colleague Henry Ezriel used in group work. What Malan added was compression, naming, and evidence, which is why the diagrams travelled under his name. The **triangle of conflict** maps the internal machinery: hidden feeling at the bottom, with anxiety and defense at the top corners, the two ways a person keeps the feeling down. The **triangle of persons** maps where that machinery runs: with past figures, usually parents, with current people in the person's life, and with the therapist in the room (Malan, 1979). One triangle for what happens inside, one for where it shows up. Together they gave therapists a real-time navigation system, and they remain the teaching backbone of every ISTDP training on earth. The next two chapters give them the full treatment.

The partnership mattered in both directions. Davanloo supplied the filmed proof that defenses could be dismantled quickly. Malan supplied the maps and the research credibility that let the discovery travel. Writing for Davanloo's own edited volume, Malan titled his contribution "The most important development in psychotherapy since the discovery of the unconscious" (Malan, 1980). Strong words from a career skeptic.

2.5 Example

Consider Cashel, a counselor seven years into practice, who attended an open evening about experiential therapies. The presenter showed a family tree: Davanloo at the root, and branching from that root, therapies Cashel had actually heard of. AEDP, with its emphasis on healing moments and positive affect, founded by Diana

Fosha, who trained in the Davanloo lineage before building her own gentler model (Fosha, 2000). Emotion-focused therapy on a nearby branch, sharing the conviction that emotional experience, not insight alone, drives change.

Cashel felt mildly cheated. He had taken an AEDP workshop two years earlier and nobody had mentioned any of this ancestry. He raised his hand and asked, a little sharply, why the family kept its relatives secret.

The presenter laughed and gave an honest answer: families quarrel. The experiential dynamic therapies share DNA and diverge hard on stance. How much pressure, how much softness, how central the therapist's warmth should be, how fast to go. The umbrella organization for these therapies, the International Experiential Dynamic Therapy Association, exists partly to keep the quarrelsome cousins at one table (International Experiential Dynamic Therapy Association, n.d.).

Cashel left the evening without picking a side, which was the right outcome. He had gained something better than an allegiance: a map of the neighborhood. When Chapter 11.0 compares these therapies properly, you will want that map too.

What this means for you: if you have brushed against AEDP, EFT, or any emotion-centered therapy, you already know some of this family. ISTDP is the intense grandparent whose discoveries the whole family inherited.

2.6 When It Doesn't Work

The most common failure with history chapters is simple: the names blur. A week from now, Davanloo, Malan, and the alphabet of descendant therapies may have merged into one vague sense of some researchers in the seventies.

That is normal. Names without anchors do not stay put, and it says nothing about your ability to learn the model itself.

Three things to try. First, keep only two names and one fact each: Davanloo filmed everything, Malan drew the triangles. That pair is genuinely all you need to proceed. Second, connect the history to something you will do, by remembering that video review exists in training because the model was born from tape. Third, if family trees help you, sketch the three-node version: Davanloo at the root, ISTDP as the trunk, AEDP and its softer cousins branching off.

If none of it sticks, skip it without guilt. History enriches understanding but does not gate it. The triangles in the next chapter will work for you no matter who invented them, and you can revisit this chapter later, when the names have faces from your own reading.

2.7 What To Take Away

ISTDP was born from a refusal and a camera. Davanloo refused to accept that deep change required years, filmed his sessions, and studied the tapes until he could see exactly how feeling rises, how anxiety discharges, and how defenses mobilize moment to moment. From that evidence he built an active method for dismantling avoidance quickly and safely. Malan, the field's great outcome researcher, supplied the two triangles that turned Davanloo's discoveries into a teachable language, and lent the enterprise scientific respectability it badly needed.

From this root grew a family of experiential dynamic therapies, including AEDP and its relatives, all sharing the conviction that experiencing avoided emotion drives change, and all arguing about how firmly to pursue it.

Two names, one fact each. Davanloo filmed everything. Malan drew the triangles. Now let's learn what he drew.

Chapter 3.0: The Triangle of Conflict

Eliora had been in session for eleven minutes when it happened, and her therapist almost missed it.

She was 29, a nurse, referred for panic attacks that had started six months earlier for no reason anyone could find. She was describing her weekend, which included a phone call from her father, who had let her know, in his mild and reasonable way, that she had chosen a disappointing career. As she reported this, three things occurred in the space of one breath. Her eyes flashed, just for an instant. Then she pulled a long sigh and rubbed her hands together as if cold. Then she said, brightly, "But honestly, he means well, and anyway, work has been so busy that I barely thought about it."

Flash. Sigh. Subject change. Eleven minutes in, Eliora had just displayed, in miniature, the entire machinery that ISTDP is built to work with. A feeling rose toward her father. Anxiety spiked in her body the instant it rose. And a defense arrived, right on schedule, to sweep the whole thing off the table.

Feeling. Anxiety. Defense. Three corners of one triangle, and this chapter teaches you to see it. By the end, you will know each corner in plain English, understand the causal chain that links them, be able to sort real client statements into the three categories, and, just as usefully, know exactly why this triangle is not the drama triangle your search results keep confusing it with. This is the single most important chapter in the book. Everything after it is application.

3.1 Three Corners in Plain English

The **triangle of conflict** is Malan's diagram of what happens inside a person when an unbearable feeling stirs (Malan, 1979). Traditionally it is drawn point-down, like a funnel. At the bottom point sits **feeling**: the true emotional response to what happened, such as anger, grief, love, longing, or joy. At the top two corners sit the forces that keep it down: **anxiety**, the alarm that fires in the body when a forbidden feeling rises, and **defense**, anything a person does to avoid experiencing the feeling.

The chain runs in one direction, and it always starts with life. Something happens: a stimulus. Your father calls. Your partner forgets. Your boss praises the colleague who did less. The stimulus evokes a feeling, welcome or not. The feeling, if it was ever punished or dangerous in your early relationships, triggers anxiety, an automatic bodily alarm. And the anxiety summons a defense, whose job is to make the feeling and the alarm go away (Frederickson, 2013).

Here is the part that changes how you sit with clients. The presenting problems that fill your intake forms, the depression, the fog, the panic, the failing relationships, are largely the visible cost of the defenses. Self-attack looks like depression. Detachment looks like emptiness. Chronic vagueness looks like confusion. The person is not broken machinery. They are running expensive machinery, and it is running exactly as designed (Frederickson, 2013).

One kindness to build in from the start: every defense was a solution first. Eliora's subject change protected a small girl who could not afford rage at the father she depended on. The solution simply outlived the problem. Hold that thought through every chapter that follows, because it is the difference between working with defenses and shaming people for them.

3.2 Why This Triangle Runs Everything

You might be thinking a diagram this simple cannot possibly guide a whole therapy. Watch what it does.

The triangle gives the ISTDP therapist a way to classify every single client response, in real time, into one of three categories. Whatever the client just did, it was feeling, anxiety, or defense. And each category has its own correct response. If feeling is present, the therapist helps the client experience it more deeply. If anxiety is too high, the therapist slows down and regulates it before going further. If a defense has arrived, the therapist helps the client see it and set it aside (Frederickson, 2013).

Assess, then respond, then assess again. Every intervention creates a new client response, which lands in one of the three corners, which tells you your next move. This loop, sometimes called moment-to-moment tracking, is the engine room of the model, and it is why trained ISTDP therapists seem uncannily responsive on video. They are not improvising brilliance. They are reading three corners and following the map (Frederickson, 2013).

The triangle also explains the model's diagnostic habit. When an ISTDP therapist meets a new client, one early question is: which defenses are producing these symptoms? A client who says "I am worthless" is not reporting a fact. Worthlessness is not a feeling; it is an activity, self-devaluation, a defense doing something to its owner. The interesting question is what feeling stirred just before the self-attack began, and toward whom (Frederickson, 2013). Chapter 6.0 takes this further. For now, notice the reflex the triangle installs: behind every symptom, look for the defense; behind every defense, look for the feeling.

3.3 Example

Meet Thibault, 44, a warehouse supervisor whose intake form said depression and low self-esteem. In his third session he described being passed over for a promotion that went to a man he had trained. His therapist asked what he felt toward his manager about that decision.

"Honestly, it makes sense," Thibault said. "I interview badly. I am not really management material. They probably saw something in him I do not have." His shoulders rounded as he spoke, and his voice went flat and dutiful.

His therapist, thinking in triangle terms, did not hear a realistic self-assessment. She heard the feeling corner slam shut and the defense corner light up. A man had been wronged, anger had presumably risen, and within two sentences the anger had been rerouted onto its owner. She said, gently, "Notice what just happened. I asked what you feel toward your manager, and you gave me three criticisms of yourself. If the criticism went where it was originally headed, toward him, what would be there?"

Thibault was quiet, and then said, with some surprise, "I trained that guy." His jaw tightened. "I trained him." It was not a volcanic moment. It was one honest degree of anger, experienced as anger, aimed at its actual target. His mood that week was slightly better; his sleep was not. The self-attack habit was decades old and did not resign after one session. But he and his therapist now shared a map: when the worthlessness talk started, they both knew to ask what feeling had just gone underground.

What this means for you: "I am worthless" is a verb wearing a noun's clothing. When self-attack appears, the triangle says a feeling toward someone else just went missing. Start listening for what vanished.

3.4 Not That Triangle

Now for the disambiguation this chapter promised, because the internet has made a genuine mess here.

Search "triangle of conflict" and you will meet two impostors. The first is the **Karpman drama triangle**, from transactional analysis, which maps three roles people play in conflicts: persecutor, rescuer, and victim (Karpman, 1968). It is a fine tool for describing interpersonal games, and it has nothing to do with Malan. Confusingly, some popular articles use "triangle of conflict" as an alternate name for Karpman's model, which is simply an error that spread. The second impostor is the Bowen family systems triangle, which describes how two people in tension recruit a third to stabilize the relationship (Bowen, 1978). Also useful. Also unrelated.

Here is the clean distinction. Karpman and Bowen describe triangles between people. Malan's triangle of conflict describes a triangle inside one person: their feeling, their anxiety, their defense (Malan, 1979). If the three corners are humans, you are not looking at Malan. If the three corners are events inside one nervous system, you are.

Why does this matter beyond trivia? Because beginners who conflate the triangles try to use Malan's model to referee relationship dynamics, and it will not do that job. Its job is psychodiagnosis: reading one person's internal response, one moment at a time. Get this distinction settled now and you will be spared the embarrassment that at least one person in every consultation group eventually suffers. It does not have to be you.

3.5 Example

Remember Keva from Chapter 1.0, the operations manager with the headaches and the bright smile? Her story shows the full triangle in motion, so let's slow the film down.

Stimulus: Sunday dinner. Her brother announces he is borrowing money from their mother again. Feeling: anger rises toward him. Keva has excellent reasons for anger; she has watched this pattern drain her mother for years. Anxiety: the instant the anger stirs, her body alarms. In Keva's case the alarm is quiet and internal, a tightening she barely registers. Defense: the smile arrives, the voice sweetens, and the sentence "I really cannot complain" performs its ancient duty.

Where does the energy go? In Keva's system, into her head. Four days a week.

In session, her therapist worked the triangle in order. First she blocked the defense, gently: "I notice you are smiling as you tell me this." Then she monitored anxiety: Keva stayed present, no fog, no panic, her body could tolerate more. Then she invited the feeling: "What is underneath the smile, toward your brother?" When the anger finally arrived weeks later, Keva described heat in her chest and an impulse in her arms, and she was startled that experiencing it felt less dangerous than a lifetime of suppressing it had.

Her outcome, you will recall, was real but partial. Fewer headaches, a brother who remained a brother. The triangle is a map of a person's inner machinery, not a lever that fixes their family.

What this means for you: try narrating one client moment this week in the four beats. Stimulus, feeling, anxiety, defense. Say nothing to the client yet. Just practice seeing the corners.

3.6 When It Doesn't Work

Here is where beginners most often stall with the triangle: everything starts looking like a defense. Your client cries and you wonder if the tears are avoidance. They get angry and you wonder if the anger is covering grief. You have gained a hammer and the world has become suspiciously full of nails, and the suspicion itself starts to poison your listening.

This happens because the categories are new, and new categories overfire. It is not a character flaw, and it fades with calibrated practice, which is exactly what training and supervision provide.

Three things to try in the meantime. First, apply the triangle to only one client, in one recorded or well-remembered moment per week, rather than running it on everyone continuously. Small doses build accuracy; constant use builds paranoia. Second, when unsure which corner you are seeing, check the body: genuine feeling tends to move through the body with energy and direction, anxiety tends to look like alarm, and defense tends to feel like something between you and the person. Third, hold your labels lightly and let the next moment correct you. The triangle is a loop, not a verdict.

And if the sorting exercise below defeats you today, leave it and return after Chapter 6.0, when defenses have their own chapter behind them. The triangle will wait.

3.7 Try the Sort

Before the summary, a small drill. Label each client statement below as feeling, anxiety, or defense. Answers follow, and getting some wrong is the point of drills.

One: "When she said that, I felt this heat come up in my chest toward her." Two: "My mind just went blank. I cannot remember what we were talking about." Three: "I suppose everyone has difficult mothers, it is hardly worth discussing." Four: "My stomach has been in knots all session." Five: "I miss him. Saying it out loud, I can feel how much." Six: "Anyway, enough about that, how are you today?" Seven: "I am probably just being dramatic about all this." Eight: "My hands are trembling right now." Nine: "I wanted to hug her. I actually wanted to hold on." Ten: "It is what it is."

Answers: one, feeling. Two, anxiety, and specifically the kind that disrupts thinking, which Chapter 5.0 will name. Three, defense, dismissal dressed as perspective. Four, anxiety. Five, feeling. Six, defense. Seven, defense, a small self-attack. Eight, anxiety. Nine, feeling, and notice it is a loving one; the triangle is not only about anger. Ten, defense, resignation in a trench coat.

Seven or more correct, excellent. Fewer, reread section 3.1 and try again tomorrow. Nobody is grading you, and calibration comes from exactly this kind of repetition.

3.8 The Short Answer

One triangle, three corners, one direction of flow. Life supplies a stimulus. The stimulus evokes a true feeling. If that feeling was dangerous in your early relationships, anxiety fires in the body the moment it rises. And a defense arrives to bury feeling and alarm together. Symptoms are largely the running cost of the defenses, which means behind every symptom you should look for the defense, and behind every defense, the missing feeling.

The triangle classifies every client response into one of three corners, and each corner has its own correct therapeutic reply: deepen feeling, regulate anxiety, or address defense. That loop guides the entire model.

And it is not the drama triangle. Karpman and Bowen map triangles between people. Malan's triangle lives inside one person. You now know the difference, permanently, which puts you ahead of half the internet.

Chapter 4.0: The Triangle of Persons

Luan's therapist realized what was happening in the fourth session, and the realization arrived as a joke.

Luan was 35, a paramedic, funny in the specific way of people whose job involves regular catastrophe. He had come to therapy because his marriage was, in his words, politely dying. Session by session, a pattern emerged in his stories. His shift supervisor was difficult, so Luan managed him with humor, kept things light, never pushed back. His wife wanted more from him emotionally, so Luan deflected with jokes until she stopped asking. His mother had been volatile his whole childhood, and young Luan had learned that a well-timed joke could sometimes redirect a storm.

In the fourth session, the therapist asked Luan what he felt about coming to therapy at all. Luan grinned and said, "Honestly, doc, this is the cheapest comedy audience I have ever had." The therapist smiled, and then did not let it pass. "Notice what you just did with me. The same move you use with your supervisor. The same move you use with your wife. The same move you learned with your mother. It just arrived here, in this room, with me."

The silence that followed was not comfortable, but it was the most honest moment of the therapy so far. Luan's oldest strategy had walked into the room and been seen.

This chapter gives you the second of Malan's two maps, the triangle of persons, which explains exactly what Luan's therapist saw and why she could use it. You will learn the three corners, what transference actually means with the mystique drained out of it, why linking the corners is how brief therapy gets its speed, and how the two triangles combine into a single navigation system.

4.1 Three Corners of People

The **triangle of persons** maps where a person's emotional patterns show up. Its corners are past figures, usually parents and early caregivers; current figures, such as partners, bosses, friends; and the therapist, right there in the room (Malan, 1979).

The claim built into the diagram is simple and enormous: the pattern is the same pattern. The machinery a person built in their earliest relationships, the specific feelings they learned to bury and the specific defenses they use to bury them, does not stay in childhood. It deploys with the boss. It deploys with the spouse. And, reliably, it deploys with the therapist, usually within the first few sessions, because therapy is exactly the kind of close, uneven, emotionally loaded relationship the machinery was built for.

Luan's humor is a clean illustration. One strategy, learned at the mother corner, running at the wife corner, the supervisor corner, and by session four, the therapist corner. Same triangle of conflict inside him each time: warm or angry feeling rises, anxiety spikes, joke deploys.

Notice what this means practically. The therapist does not have to rely on the client's reports about their life, which are filtered through the very defenses in question. The pattern performs itself live, in the room, available for direct observation. Malan's two triangles, used together, let the therapist watch the internal machinery (triangle of conflict) and track its address (triangle of persons) at the same time (Malan, 1979).

4.2 Transference Without the Mystique

Transference is one of those words that makes sensible clinicians roll their eyes, so let's strip it down. Transference means responding to a present person with feelings, expectations, and strategies that were built for a past one. That is the whole concept. If you have ever flinched at a boss's neutral email because your father communicated in neutral-seeming ambushes, you have experienced it. Nothing spooky is occurring. Old learning is generalizing, which is what learning does.

What makes ISTDP distinctive is not believing in transference. Most therapies do, in some vocabulary. It is how actively the model uses it. Because the client's core pattern arrives in the room and aims itself at the therapist, the therapist can work with the live pattern rather than descriptions of it. When Luan jokes at his therapist, she does not need a history lesson; the history is currently happening to her.

There is a deeper layer, which you will meet again in Chapters 8.0 and 10.0. Davanloo observed that when a therapist blocks a client's defenses and keeps inviting real feeling, something rises in the client toward the therapist: a compound of irritation at being pressed, fear, guilt, and underneath it, often, hope and something like love, because someone is finally refusing to be fended off. He called this mixture complex transference feelings, and he found that when it rises high enough, it acts like a key: the old buried feelings toward the original figures surge up with it, and the past becomes directly available (Davanloo, 1990). For now, do not worry about mastering that. Just register that in this model, what the client feels toward the therapist is not a complication in the work. It is the work arriving.

4.3 Example

Meet Mehreen, 47, a project director who came to therapy after her third consecutive relationship ended the same way: the partner complained she was never really there. In early sessions she was impeccable. Prepared, articulate, faintly managerial. She answered every question fully and revealed nothing.

Around session six, her therapist tried a linking observation. "Can I share a pattern I think I see? You have told me your father demanded performance and had no patience for needs. You have told me your partners eventually felt shut out behind your competence. And I notice that with me, you arrive with an agenda, brief me thoroughly, and steer us away any time something unrehearsed starts to happen. Past, present, and here. Does that fit?"

Mehreen's first response was to manage the observation. She agreed it was an interesting hypothesis and offered to think about it, which both of them noticed was the pattern performing itself again, and they laughed, and the laugh cracked something open. What came through the crack was not dramatic. It was a small, unrehearsed sentence: "If I stop performing, I do not know what I am for."

The therapy did not become easy after that. Mehreen canceled two of the next four sessions, competence reasserting itself as scheduling. But the link had been made, and it held. When she managed, they could both name it, and increasingly she could feel the loneliness underneath the management, which was the feeling the whole system existed to avoid.

What this means for you: a linking observation joins at least two corners of the triangle of persons, ideally including the room. It converts a lifetime pattern from biography into live experience, which is the only place it can change.

4.4 Why Linking Creates Speed

Here is the engineering explanation for why brief dynamic therapy can be brief at all, and it comes straight from Malan's research.

In open-ended therapy, insight often stays regional. The client understands their childhood in the childhood conversations, complains about their marriage in the marriage conversations, and relates to the therapist in a third register entirely, with nothing connecting the rooms. Change under those conditions is slow because the learning does not transfer.

Malan's outcome studies pointed at something specific: interpretations that linked the corners, particularly ones connecting the pattern with the therapist to the pattern with parents, were associated with better results (Malan, 1979). Later work in the Davanloo tradition treats the full link, past figure to current figure to therapist, as a central lever of the method (Malan & Coughlin Della Selva, 2006). Every time the triangle closes, the client experiences, rather than merely concludes, that it is one pattern, one set of buried feelings, one machinery, wearing different faces. That single realization does the work that years of regional insight might not.

There is a humbling implication for you as a future practitioner. To link the corners, you must be willing to be a corner. The moments when the client's pattern lands on you, bores you, charms you, manages you, pushes you away, are not interruptions of the therapy. They are the material. Learning to notice what a client evokes in you, without acting on it or taking it personally, is a trainable skill, and Chapter 12.0 will tell you where it gets trained.

4.5 Example

One more, because the triangle of persons also runs on positive feeling, and beginners forget that.

Meet Yonatan, 61, retired, who sought therapy after his wife's death. His grief was real and he could touch it. What he could not touch, he discovered, was gratitude. In session nine, his therapist made a simple, warm observation about how hard Yonatan had worked between sessions. Yonatan's eyes filled, and then, in the space of a breath, he made a small dismissive gesture and said the therapist was paid to say that.

His therapist stayed with it. "Something happened just now. I said something kind, something rose in you, and you swatted it away. Who taught you that kindness has a catch?" The answer reached back fifty years, to a household where affection was scarce and usually invoiced. Warmth from his wife had been tolerable only in small doses, a fact he now grieved doubly.

Notice the triangle: therapist corner (the compliment), past corner (the invoicing household), current corner (the marriage where he rationed the love he received). And notice the feeling being defended against was love, not rage. The triangle of conflict at the bottom of all this had longing and tenderness at its feeling corner. ISTDP is often caricatured as anger archaeology, and the caricature misses this: some of the most defended feelings in any caseload are the warm ones (Frederickson, 2013).

What this means for you: when a client deflects your warmth, waves off praise, or cannot receive care, you are watching the triangle of persons operate on positive affect. It deserves the same gentle attention as any defense.

4.6 When It Doesn't Work

The classic beginner failure with this material is the premature link. You spot a gorgeous parallel between the client's father and their reaction to you, you deliver it with a flourish in session three, and the client looks at you as if you have started speaking Elvish. Or worse, they politely agree, file it away, and nothing changes.

Why it goes wrong: links only land when the feeling is warm on the table. A pattern pointed out intellectually is just an interesting fact; a pattern caught in the act, while the client can still feel the impulse behind it, is an experience. Timing is most of the craft, and timing is precisely what beginners do not have yet. That is not an insult. It is a definition.

Three things to try. First, collect links privately before you ever speak one. Write the three corners for one client and watch for a week; observation without intervention is legitimate practice. Second, when you do share a pattern, offer it as a question with an escape hatch, the way Mehreen's therapist did: does that fit? Third, anchor every link in something that happened in the room within the last two minutes, not in theory.

If linking feels beyond you entirely right now, good. Noticing that is accurate self-assessment, and the skill lives in supervised training, where it belongs. Watching the corners is your work for now, and it is real work.

4.7 Pulling It Together

You now hold both of Malan's maps. The triangle of conflict runs inside the person: feeling, anxiety, defense, in that order, with symptoms as the running cost. The triangle of persons tracks where that machinery deploys: with past figures who installed it, with current figures who trigger it, and with the therapist, on whom it reliably lands within a few sessions.

Transference, stripped of mystique, is old learning generalizing to a new person, and ISTDP treats its arrival in the room as the material of the work rather than a nuisance. Linking the corners, especially connecting what happens with the therapist to where it began, converts biography into live experience, and Malan's research suggests those links are a genuine engine of brief therapy's speed.

Two triangles, one system. Inside, and where. From here on, the book teaches you to read them in motion, starting with the corner beginners fear most: anxiety, and the three doors it leaves the body through.

Chapter 5.0: How Anxiety Shows Up

Delyth will tell you about the session herself, because she tells every new trainee she meets, as a public service.

Two years into practice, she had read enough about emotion-focused work to be dangerous. A client named Tovey, 33, was describing his father's drinking, and Delyth, sensing buried anger, leaned in and pressed. What do you feel toward him? What is happening in your body? Stay with it. She was doing, she believed, the intense kind of therapy.

Tovey's answers got shorter. Then slower. Then he said, "Sorry, what was the question?" His eyes had gone distant, his face slack, and when Delyth asked what he was aware of, he said, from somewhere far away, "The room looks kind of flat. Like a photo of a room."

Delyth felt a cold drop in her stomach. Whatever was happening, it was not a breakthrough. She backed off, talked gently about the weekend, and Tovey slowly returned to the room. She spent that evening searching for what she had seen, and found it in the ISTDP literature within an hour: cognitive-perceptual disruption. The third pathway. The stop signal. She had been flooring the accelerator of a car whose engine was already hydrolocking.

This chapter teaches you what Delyth learned the hard way. Anxiety is not one thing. In this model it is a bodily discharge with three distinct channels, each one visible if you know where to look, and each one carrying a different instruction for the therapist. By the end you will know all three patterns, what each means for pacing, why this is the model's central safety skill, and how to start observing without intervening.

5.1 Watching the Body First

Here is the shift this chapter asks of you: in ISTDP, anxiety is something you watch, not only something the client reports.

The reasoning goes back to the triangle of conflict. When a forbidden feeling rises, anxiety fires automatically, in the body, before and often instead of any conscious report. Clients frequently do not know they are anxious; their bodies announce it anyway. Davanloo, reviewing thousands of hours of tape, observed that this bodily discharge is not random. It runs down specific physiological channels, and which channel is active tells you something crucial: how much rising feeling this person's system can currently tolerate (Davanloo, 1990).

That last sentence is why ISTDP therapists watch hands, breath, and eyes the way pilots watch instruments. The channels are a live readout of capacity. The literature describes the therapist calibrating pressure to what the patient's system can bear, and the channels are how you know what it can bear (ten Have-de Labije & Neborsky, 2012). Read them correctly and the work stays challenging but safe. Read them wrong, as Delyth did, and you are pressing feeling on a system that has already run out of room.

A quick reassurance before the three patterns, because this is where non-medical readers tense up. You do not need physiology training. Every sign described below is visible from a chair, with no equipment beyond attention. Thousands of talk-trained therapists have learned this grammar. The vocabulary sounds anatomical; the skill is observational.

5.2 The First Pathway

The first channel is discharge into the **striated muscles**, the voluntary muscles of the arms, legs, chest, and jaw. This is the pattern you already know from ordinary life: tension.

What you see from your chair: the client sighs, and keeps sighing, big involuntary breaths that punctuate the conversation.

Hands clench and unclench, or grip the chair. Arms cross tightly. The jaw sets. Shoulders climb. The client may report tension or restlessness if asked, but the body has already told you.

Here is the counterintuitive part, and it is the most practically useful fact in this chapter: in this model, striated discharge is broadly a green light. It means feeling is rising and the person's system is containing it in the muscles, the healthiest and most mature of the three channels. The sighing client is a client whose unconscious is engaged and whose capacity is holding (Abbass, 2015). Trained therapists see a deep sigh after a pressing question and are quietly encouraged. The work is working.

Green light does not mean floor it. It means the current pace is tolerable, and rising feeling should continue to be invited while you keep watching. Anxiety patterns can shift within a single session, which is why the watching never stops.

Try this reframe on your own material this week: the next time a client sighs heavily while approaching something difficult, silently note it not as distress to be soothed away but as evidence of feeling on the move. You do not have to do anything differently yet. Just recategorize the sigh.

5.3 The Second Pathway

The second channel is discharge into the **smooth muscles**, the involuntary muscles of the gut, blood vessels, and airways. When anxiety runs down this channel, it stops looking like tension and starts looking like illness.

What you see, or more often hear about: the stomach knots, churns, or cramps. Nausea arrives mid-session. The client mentions irritable bowel symptoms, migraines, sudden urgency to use the bathroom, or feeling suddenly exhausted and drained. The tension signs of the first pathway may be strangely absent; the client can look calm while their gut riots.

The meaning is different and the instruction is different. Smooth muscle discharge signals that rising feeling has exceeded what the striated system can hold, and the overflow is going internal. It is a slow-down signal: the therapist's job shifts from inviting more feeling to regulating anxiety first, helping the client notice and name what is happening in their body until the discharge returns to the striated channel, and only then proceeding (ten Have-de Labije & Neborsky, 2012).

There is a larger clinical payoff hiding here. A substantial body of research links emotional processes to medically unexplained physical symptoms, and short-term dynamic therapy has meaningful evidence for helping somatic conditions (Abbass, Kisely, & Kroenke, 2009). Keva's headaches from Chapter 1.0 were this pathway wearing a symptom's face. Once you know this channel exists, a certain kind of mystery patient, scanned, tested, and cleared by every specialist in town, becomes legible.

5.4 The Third Pathway

The third channel is not really a discharge into the body at all. It is a disruption of the mind's instruments, and the field calls it **cognitive-perceptual disruption**.

What you see is what Delyth saw in Tovey. Thinking fogs. The client loses the thread mid-sentence, asks what the question was, goes blank. Perception distorts: vision blurs or flattens, sounds recede, the room turns unreal or photo-like. The client may drift somewhere far away, and dissociative language appears: floaty, not really here, watching myself from outside.

This is the stop signal, full stop. It means anxiety has overwhelmed the channels that could contain it and is now disrupting the machinery of thought and perception itself. Pressing feeling into this state does not produce breakthrough; it produces flooding, fragmentation, and a client who learns that therapy is somewhere they go to feel unsafe. The correct response is immediate anxiety regulation: stop the exploration, bring the client back to the present, engage their thinking with simple concrete attention to what is happening in their body, and do not resume feeling-work in that session unless the system fully settles (Frederickson, 2013).

Clients whose anxiety habitually runs down this third channel, or the second, at low levels of feeling need a fundamentally adapted approach. That approach exists, it is called the graded format, and Chapter 9.0 is devoted to it. For now, the rule for you is simpler and absolute: fog means stop. If you learn one safety rule from this entire book, make it that one.

5.5 Example

Watch all three channels move through one composite session.

Bintou, 41, sought therapy about her mother, recently diagnosed with dementia. Early in the session, describing the diagnosis appointment, she sighed repeatedly, deep chest-lifting sighs, and her hands worked in her lap. Striated. Her therapist, reading green, gently invited more: "A lot is rising as you describe that room. What is the feeling toward your mother, underneath the sadness?"

Complicated feeling stirred, guilt and anger braided together, the kind adult children of declining parents know well. Bintou's sighing stopped. She mentioned, almost in passing, that her stomach had gone into a knot and she suddenly felt carsick. Smooth muscle. The therapist shifted without fanfare: "Let's pause the story. Notice the stomach. Where exactly is the knot? Just describe it." They spent four unhurried minutes on the plain sensations, and the nausea eased, and a long sigh returned. Striated again. The system had made room.

Only then did the therapist reopen the door, more gently: "There was anger arriving toward your mother before your stomach interrupted. Some part of you may feel it is not allowed. Can we look at it together?" This time the feeling came through the muscles: jaw tight, fists closing, and then words Bintou had never permitted herself about years of being her mother's unpaid keeper.

No fog appeared at any point; had it appeared, the session would have changed course entirely. Bintou left tired and lighter. The guilt about her anger did not disappear that day, and honestly it never disappeared completely. It became discussable, which was enough to build on.

What this means for you: the channels are not a diagnosis of a person; they are a weather report, updated minute by minute, and the therapist's pacing follows the weather.

5.6 Example

Return to Delyth and Tovey, because the story continues and the continuation matters.

After the flat-photo session, Delyth did three things right. She stopped pressing feeling with Tovey entirely. She sought consultation with a supervisor who knew the model. And in the next session, she repaired: she told Tovey, plainly, that she had pushed too hard the previous week, that his fogging out was his system protecting him and not a failure, and that they would go slower.

Tovey's response taught her as much as the fog had. He said no therapist had ever told him the spacing-out had a name. He had assumed, since childhood, that it meant something was deeply wrong with his brain. The psychoeducation alone, that this was anxiety taking a particular exit, and that it could change, visibly moved him. It was striated movement, a sigh, the first she had ever seen from him.

Under supervision, Delyth learned the graded approach you will meet in Chapter 9.0, and worked with Tovey in small, titrated steps:

a little feeling, then attention to the body, then thinking about what they had noticed together. Progress was real and slow. Eight months in, Tovey could feel irritation toward his father for nearly a minute before the fog gathered, and he could tell Delyth the fog was starting, which changed everything about their pacing. He was not finished. He was, for the first time, on a road.

What this means for you: misreading the channels is survivable if you notice, back off, repair, and get supervision. The unforgivable version is the one where the therapist never learns the signs at all.

5.7 When It Doesn't Work

The predictable failure with this chapter is sign-hunting paralysis. You sit with your next client silently chanting striated, smooth, fog, miss half of what they say, and end the session having watched their hands so intently you forgot to be a person with them.

This is what happens when observation is new: it consumes the attention it will later run on for free. Every driver stared at the gearstick once.

Three things to try. First, watch for one channel per week, not three. Week one, only sighs and muscle tension. Week two, only somatic complaints. Week three, only fog. Stacking them comes later and comes naturally. Second, use recordings if you have them, or process notes written immediately after session, so live attention is not carrying the whole load. Third, borrow a habit from training programs and watch published demonstration videos with the sound off for five minutes, just reading bodies. The signal is easier to see when the words are not competing.

And if body-watching genuinely is not landing yet, set it down. Read Chapters 6.0 through 8.0, where the defenses and the therapist's stance give the channels their context, then return. This chapter improves on the second visit more than any other in the book.

5.8 Before You Move On

Anxiety in this model is a bodily discharge with three channels, and the active channel is a live readout of how much rising feeling the person's system can hold. Striated muscle discharge, the sighing, clenching, tension pattern, is broadly a green light: feeling is rising and capacity is holding. Smooth muscle discharge, the gut-and-migraine pattern, is a slow-down signal: regulate anxiety first, then proceed. Cognitive-perceptual disruption, the fog, blankness, and unreality pattern, is a stop signal, always, no exceptions worth learning as a beginner.

Watching is a skill that costs attention now and becomes free later. Build it one channel at a time, on one client at a time, and let fog means stop settle into your bones before anything else.

You can now read the alarm system. Next, the machinery it protects: the defenses themselves.

Chapter 6.0: Meeting the Defenses

Anthoula arrived at her first session with a folder.

She was 39, a policy analyst, and the folder contained a typed summary of her childhood, organized by theme, with a page of hypotheses about the origins of her difficulties. She handed it across and said, "I thought this would save us time." Her difficulties, the folder explained, included an inability to sustain intimate relationships, which she attributed, with footnoted precision, to an emotionally unavailable father and a critical mother.

Her therapist read the first page, genuinely impressed, and then set the folder down and asked a question that was not in it. "As you sit here, handing your childhood to a stranger in a folder, what do you feel?"

Anthoula began to answer with a theory about her attachment style. The therapist smiled gently. "That is what you think. I asked what you feel." A longer pause. "I feel," Anthoula said slowly, "like you just took away my folder." And for one unguarded second, she looked exactly as frightened as a person meeting a stranger without armor, which is what she was.

The folder was a defense. A magnificent one, decades in the making, polished into a professional asset and a personality. This chapter is about defenses: what they are, the common cast you will meet in any caseload, the crucial distinction between the quick ones and the load-bearing ones, and how ISTDP helps people see their own armor without ever being shamed for wearing it.

6.1 Old Solutions Still Running

A **defense** is anything a person does, inside or outside awareness, to avoid experiencing a feeling. That definition is deliberately wide. Changing the subject is a defense. So is explaining instead of feeling, joking, going vague, attacking yourself, going numb, staying impressively busy, and handing your therapist a folder.

The compassionate frame from Chapter 3.0 bears repeating, because it is the difference between this work and criticism. Every defense was a solution first. A child in a home where anger got you punished, or where tears got you mocked, or where needs got you abandoned, faced an engineering problem: how to keep having a nervous system in an environment that punished its output. Defenses were the engineering. They were adaptive, often brilliant, and at the time, genuinely necessary (Coughlin Della Selva, 2004).

The trouble is that the machinery does not check the calendar. Anthoula's intellectualizing protected a girl whose feelings were treated as errors. Forty years later the danger is gone, the machinery runs on, and the maintenance bill has come due as loneliness. In the model's blunt accounting, from Chapter 3.0: symptoms and presenting problems are largely caused by defenses, which means the defenses, not the childhood stories about them, are the working target of the therapy (Frederickson, 2012).

One more reframe before the field guide. Defenses are not who the person is. They are things the person does, and this distinction is not philosophical garnish. Doing implies the possibility of not doing. The whole therapy runs through that gap.

6.2 The Common Cast

You will meet the same defenses so often that they deserve introductions, like recurring characters in a long series.

Intellectualization turns feeling into analysis. Anthoula's folder; Orson's castle tour from Chapter 1.0. The client discusses their rage the way a critic discusses a film they did not much like. **Vagueness** dissolves specifics into mist: things have been hard lately, it is all a bit much, you know how it is. Feelings live in specific moments, so vagueness starves them of habitat.

Rationalization supplies reasonable-sounding cover: he means well, everyone has difficult mothers, it makes sense they promoted the other guy. **Humor**, Luan's specialty from Chapter 4.0, discharges the tension of a rising feeling as a laugh before the feeling can land. **Detachment** simply unplugs: the flat voice, the shrug, the it-is-what-it-is. And **self-attack**, Thibault's pattern from Chapter 3.0, reroutes feeling meant for someone else back onto its owner, which is among the most symptom-productive defenses in the catalog, strongly tied to depression in this model's account (Frederickson, 2013).

Notice something about this cast: every one of them is socially rewarded somewhere. Intellectualizers get promoted. Humorists get invited to parties. Detached people get praised as low-maintenance. Self-attackers get called humble. Defenses persist not only because they mute feeling but because the world often pays people to keep them, which is worth remembering the next time surrendering one proves hard.

You might be thinking that you recognized yourself at least twice in that paragraph. Of course you did. Everyone runs defenses; the difference is degree, cost, and flexibility. Therapists are not exempt, and Chapter 12.0 will have more to say about what happens when your own favorites meet a training camera.

6.3 Quick Moves and Load Bearing Walls

The field draws a distinction you should have in place early, between tactical defenses and character defenses.

Tactical defenses are the quick moves, deployed in the moment, mostly at the surface of contact between two people. The subject change. The little laugh. The "I suppose" and "sort of" and "maybe" that dilute every statement. The answering of a different question than the one asked. They are the pawns of the defensive system:

numerous, mobile, individually cheap (ten Have-de Labije & Neborsky, 2012).

Character defenses are the load-bearing walls. These are defenses so long-running that they have been mistaken, by everyone including their owner, for personality. Anthoula is not a woman who sometimes intellectualizes; she has built a self out of it. The lifelong pleaser. The permanently reasonable man. The one who never needs anything. Character defenses do not deploy in the moment because they never switch off (Coughlin Della Selva, 2004).

Why the distinction matters: they are worked with differently, and they signal differently. Tactical defenses can often simply be noticed and set aside, and a motivated client learns to catch their own within weeks. Character defenses require patient, repeated work, because dismantling one feels to the client like demolition of the self, and in a sense they are right. The person who stops pleasing must discover what they are when nobody is being pleased, and there is grief in that discovery, not just liberation.

For you, at this stage, the distinction is observational. When you spot avoidance, ask yourself quietly: was that a move, or is that the architecture?

6.4 Example

Watch the difference between pointing at a defense and shaming a person, because the entire craft lives in that difference.

Meet Raha, 26, a graduate student whose relationships kept ending at the three-month mark. In session, describing the most recent ending, she shrugged and said, "It is fine. He was too attached anyway. I do not really do feelings, it is kind of my brand."

A shaming response, and beginners produce these accidentally, would be: "You use detachment to push people away, and that is why you are alone." Every word arguably true, and the client leaves smaller, defended harder, and probably does not come back.

Her actual therapist did something structurally different. First, she made the defense visible as an action: "Can I point at something? A moment ago, when you mentioned him crying at the end, something crossed your face. Then the shrug arrived, and 'it is fine,' and the brand. The shrug seems to be doing a job." Then she honored its history: "I would guess the shrug has protected you for a long time, and that it earned its keep somewhere." Then, the move that defines the model, she pointed at the cost and put the choice in Raha's hands: "The trouble is what it costs you now. It ends your relationships at three months, and it is currently keeping me at the same distance. So we have a real choice here. We can honor the shrug and stay comfortable, or we can look at what it is guarding. Which do you want?"

Raha, to her own surprise, said quietly, "Nobody ever asked." What was under the shrug took months to reach and turned out to be an old and simple terror of being left first. The three-month pattern, she and her therapist eventually mapped, was Raha firing people before they could resign. Her next relationship ended at five months, ended by the other person, and Raha grieved it properly, which she rated, accurately, as progress.

What this means for you: the sequence is the skill. See the defense as an action, honor its history, name its present cost, and hand the choice back. Judgment appears nowhere in the sequence.

6.5 Example

One defense deserves special handling, and Cashel, the counselor from Chapter 2.0, met it from the client's chair.

Cashel entered personal therapy during his own training, mostly out of curiosity. He was, you will recall, funny. His therapist enjoyed him for two sessions and then, in the third, after a joke about his father's funeral got a laugh, said something Cashel still quotes. "You are genuinely funny. And I notice the jokes arrive exactly when something starts to hurt. I laugh, you get relief, and the hurt goes back in the drawer. I do not want to keep taking that deal at your expense."

Cashel's first response was, naturally, another joke. His therapist smiled and waited. What followed was the strangest silence of Cashel's adult life, in which he discovered he had almost no idea how to be in a room, unfunny, with another person, and that under the performance was a boy whose humor had been the only reliable way to make a depressed parent's face change.

Here is the honest outcome. Cashel did not stop being funny, and the therapy never asked him to. What changed was flexibility. The humor became a choice rather than a reflex, something he could set down when closeness mattered. His wife noticed before he did. Some sessions he still joked his way through, and his therapist would name the deal on the table, and sometimes Cashel took the deal anyway. Defenses do not surrender; they loosen.

What this means for you: the goal of defense work is never amputation. It is flexibility, the restored ability to choose. Clients keep their humor, their competence, their analysis. They just stop being run by them.

6.6 When It Doesn't Work

The signature beginner failure with defenses is the accidental prosecution. You learn the vocabulary, start spotting defenses accurately, and your observations begin arriving with a faint but unmistakable flavor of gotcha. Clients feel caught rather than seen, comply rather than open, or politely stop coming.

Why it happens: naming defenses feels powerful, and power is intoxicating exactly in proportion to how new it is. Also, honestly, some of us were drawn to this field by our own inner critics, and a defense-spotting framework offers that critic a professional license.

Three things to try. First, install the two-part rule: never name a cost without first honoring the history. "This protected you" comes before "this is costing you," every time, in that order. Second, check your inner tone before speaking: if the observation feels like winning, do not say it yet. Third, run the frame on yourself weekly. Catch one of your own defenses, notice how it feels to be caught, and let that feeling calibrate your touch with clients.

And permission, because this one matters: you are allowed to spot defenses for months without naming any of them aloud. Silent accurate observation is not cowardice. It is the correct first stage of a skill whose second stage belongs in supervision.

6.7 The Heart of It

A defense is anything a person does to avoid experiencing a feeling, and every defense was a solution before it was a problem. The common cast, intellectualization, vagueness, rationalization, humor, detachment, self-attack, persists because it works, and because the world often rewards it. Tactical defenses are moves; character defenses are architecture mistaken for personality, and the two are worked with differently.

The craft of defense work is a sequence with judgment nowhere in it: make the defense visible as an action, honor what it once protected, name what it costs now, and hand the choice back to its owner. The goal is never to strip a person of their armor but to return the armor to their control.

You can now see the machinery and read its alarm system. The next chapter puts both skills in motion where every therapy starts: the first session.

Chapter 7.0: The First Session

Ledger booked the appointment on a Tuesday and spent the following week rehearsing.

He was 48, a building contractor, and he had done therapy twice before. He knew the drill, or believed he did. You describe your childhood in the first session, your symptoms in the second, and then you circle the airport indefinitely. He had prepared a tidy narrative: divorced, drinking more than he liked, probably work stress, mother difficult, next question.

Carwen, his new therapist, did not follow the script. Ninety seconds of pleasantries, and then: "So that we use your time well, tell me the problem you most want help with. Not the whole story yet. The problem, in a sentence." Ledger opened with the rehearsed material, and Carwen listened, and then asked something no intake had ever asked him. "When was the last specific time this problem showed up? Walk me through that moment. Where were you standing? What happened first?"

Ledger, mildly annoyed, described the previous Friday: his ex-wife's text about their daughter's school fees, the third whiskey, the hollow evening. As he talked, he heard his own voice change. The rehearsed narrative had been about a man with problems. This was just Friday, and Friday, it turned out, had feelings in it. Twenty minutes into his third attempt at therapy, Ledger said, "Nobody has ever asked me about an actual day before," and meant it as a complaint, and noticed it was not one.

This chapter walks you through what Carwen was doing. The ISTDP first session has a structure, a purpose, and a name for its parts: inquiry, psychodiagnosis, and the building of a focus and an alliance. By the end you will understand each part, see why the model treats assessment as something you do by working rather than before working, and be able to upgrade your own opening questions immediately, no training required.

7.1 Inquiry Means Specifics

The first phase of an ISTDP session is **dynamic inquiry**: an active, specific exploration of the problem the person wants help with, at the level of concrete moments rather than summaries (Lied, 2025).

The word active is doing real work. The therapist is not a receptionist for whatever material happens to arrive. They pursue: what is the problem, when did it last occur, what happened, what did you feel, what did you do. And the word specific is doing even more. Feelings, as section 6.2 noted, live in specific moments. Summaries are where they go to die. "My marriage is struggling" contains no feeling. "On Friday she texted about the school fees and I poured a third whiskey" is made of feeling, lightly buried.

There is a diagnostic reason for the specificity too. Vagueness, remember, is a defense, one of the most common in the deck. A client who cannot produce a single concrete example of their own problem is showing you, in the first ten minutes, exactly how their avoidance operates. That is not a failed inquiry. That is data (Frederickson, 2013).

Beginners sometimes worry the specificity is cold, an interrogation. Watch the tapes and you find the opposite: clients like Ledger experience it as the first evidence anyone intends to actually help. There is a particular relief in being asked about Friday by someone who plainly plans to do something with the answer. Declining to waste a person's time is a form of respect, and clients feel it as one.

7.2 Watching While Asking

The second thing happening in an ISTDP first session is invisible to the client, and it is the reason this book made you read Chapters 3.0 through 6.0 first. While the therapist inquires, they watch. Every question is also a probe, and every response gets read against the triangle of conflict: did feeling rise, did anxiety fire, and if so down which channel, did a defense arrive, and which one. The field calls this running assessment **psychodiagnosis**, and it is happening continuously from the first minute (ten Have-de Labije & Neborsky, 2012).

This is the model's answer to a question you may not have thought to ask: where is the assessment phase? Most training teaches assessment as a separate activity, a form-filling fortnight before therapy proper begins. ISTDP collapses the distinction. You assess by beginning, because the only way to learn how a person's system responds to rising feeling is to invite a little rising feeling and watch. Davanloo's name for the extended first encounter was the trial therapy: a first session, often a long one, that is simultaneously a genuine attempt to help and a live test of what this particular nervous system does under emotional load (Davanloo, 1990).

What the watching yields is a working answer to the questions that set the entire treatment's course. Where does this person's anxiety discharge, striated, smooth, or fog? Which defenses come, and are they moves or architecture? And, summing those, how much capacity does this system have, which determines from the very first session which road the therapy takes: the standard route, or the graded one that Chapter 9.0 describes.

The decision logic, once the reading is made, is the one you already know from section 3.2: feeling gets deepened, excessive anxiety gets regulated, defense gets addressed (Frederickson, 2012). First sessions differ from later ones only in how much of the map is still blank.

7.3 Example

Return to Carwen and Ledger, because their first session illustrates the loop in motion.

When Ledger described Friday, feeling stirred visibly: his jaw worked as he mentioned the text, and a long sigh escaped as he described pouring the drink. Striated discharge, capacity holding. Carwen, reading green, went one step further in. "When her text arrived, before the whiskey. What was the feeling toward her, right then?"

Ledger's system answered before Ledger did. "Ah, you know," he said, waving a hand, "she is doing her best. Money is genuinely tight. It is what it is." Rationalization, then resignation, two defenses in nine seconds. And here is the part worth studying: Carwen did not bulldoze them, in a first session, with the alliance twenty minutes old. She made them visible and recruited Ledger against them instead. "Notice what just happened. I asked what you felt toward her, and you defended her twice and then shrugged. If we let the shrug run this therapy, we will have a very polite year and your Fridays will not change. What do you actually feel when that text lands?"

Ledger laughed, once, without humor, and said, "Furious. I feel furious, and then I feel like garbage for being furious, because she is right about the money." In one sentence: feeling, and the self-attack that punishes it. Carwen now had a triangle sketch of Ledger's system, drawn from live data, twenty-five minutes into their acquaintance.

The session did not produce a breakthrough, and Carwen was not hunting one. It produced something more valuable for a first session: an accurate map and a client who had experienced, rather than been told, what the work would be like.

What this means for you: notice that every therapeutic move in that room was also an assessment move. That fusion, helping as testing, testing as helping, is the signature of the model's opening.

7.4 Building the Alliance

The third strand of the first session is the one that makes the other two survivable: the conscious building of a working alliance around an agreed task.

ISTDP is demanding, and the model is clear-eyed about this. No one can be pressed toward their most avoided feelings by a stranger and tolerate it unless they understand why it is happening and have signed up for it. So the therapist works, explicitly, to establish three agreements: what we are here to change (the goal), how we will work on it together (the task), and the felt sense that the therapist is an ally in the struggle rather than its author (Lied, 2025).

In practice this sounds unglamorous. It sounds like Carwen saying: "So the pattern seems to be, fury arrives, you turn it on yourself, and the whiskey handles the wreckage. Is that the thing you want us to change?" And Ledger saying yes. And Carwen continuing: "Then here is what working on it will involve. When the fury shows up in here, and it will, my job is to help you feel it rather than shrug it off or drink it later. That will sometimes be uncomfortable. Do you want that from me?" And Ledger, after a genuine pause, saying yes to that too.

That exchange looks small. It is load-bearing. Every difficult moment later in the therapy stands on it, because when Ledger's defenses rise against Carwen, as Chapter 4.0 promised they will, she can appeal to an agreement Ledger himself made: you asked me not to take the shrug for an answer. The client's own healthy will, recruited early and explicitly, is what the therapist works with rather than against. Without it, pressure is just pressure. With it, pressure is a promise being kept (Frederickson, 2013).

7.5 Example

Not every first session goes like Ledger's, and you should watch one that went sideways.

Sama, a newly qualified therapist, was so taken with dynamic inquiry after a workshop that she ran it at full intensity with her very next intake, a 52-year-old client named Firdous who had come in describing panic attacks and a recent redundancy. Sama pursued specifics briskly: last panic attack, walk me through it, what did you feel, what came before. Good questions, wrong dosage. She was inquiring; she was not watching.

Fifteen minutes in, Firdous mentioned her chest going tight and her thoughts turning to syrup, and asked, apologetically, if they could open a window. Sama, intent on her next question, said in a moment. Two questions later, Firdous had gone quiet and vague, answering in fragments, eyes fixed on the carpet. The session limped to its end, and Firdous did not book a second.

In supervision, the recording told the story Sama had missed live. The tightening chest and syrupy thinking had been the second and third channels announcing themselves early, a system with limited capacity asking for regulation, and the request for a window had practically been a flare. Firdous had needed the pace slowed and her anxiety attended to, and instead received three more excellent questions.

Sama's supervisor was kind about it, and precise: the questions were fine; the failure was that inquiry had outrun psychodiagnosis. Asking without watching is not ISTDP, just interrogation with better intentions. Sama wrote the line on a card above her desk. There was no repair to make with Firdous, who never returned, and Sama had to metabolize that too, because this work has real stakes and not every lesson refunds its tuition.

What this means for you: the two strands are a braid, not a sequence. If you upgrade your questions after this chapter, upgrade your watching in the same breath, and let the watching set the pace.

7.6 When It Doesn't Work

Here is how this chapter typically fails in practice: you try specific inquiry with a real client, and the client cannot do it. You ask for one concrete example and receive fog, or a decade-spanning summary, or "I cannot really think of one," and you conclude the method does not work on your caseload.

Reframe it. The method just worked. A person who cannot retrieve a single specific instance of their own presenting problem has shown you their defensive system operating at the level of memory and attention itself, which is significant information about capacity and often a sign the graded road of Chapter 9.0 is the right one. Nothing failed; something got measured.

Three things to try. First, shrink the ask: not the last time the problem occurred, but simply this morning, walked through hour by hour. Almost everyone can do this morning, and problems have a way of appearing in it. Second, offer a menu instead of an open field: was there a moment this week with your partner, at work, with your body? Choices retrieve better than blank prompts. Third, if all specifics keep dissolving, stop pursuing and name the pattern warmly: I notice specifics are hard to hold onto, and that is worth understanding together, because it is probably part of the picture.

And if you try the upgraded questions for two weeks and feel clumsy, that is the correct feeling. Carwen has asked those questions several thousand times. You are allowed to be visibly new at this.

7.7 In Plain Terms

An ISTDP first session braids three strands. Dynamic inquiry pursues the problem in concrete, specific moments, because feelings live in Fridays, not in summaries, and because a client's difficulty producing specifics is itself diagnostic. Psychodiagnosis runs continuously underneath: every response is read against the triangle, anxiety channels are tracked, defenses are cataloged, and the person's capacity determines which road the therapy takes. And the alliance is built consciously and out loud, around explicit agreement on the goal and the task, so that every hard moment later stands on the client's own stated will.

Assessment, in this model, is not a phase before the work. It is the work, watched carefully. And the two strands must move together, because inquiry without watching is interrogation.

You have now seen the opening. The next chapter faces the question you have been carrying since the Introduction: what about the pressure, and is this model as aggressive as its reputation?

Chapter 8.0: Pressure Without Pushing

Ozias watched the training video with his arms folded, waiting to be appalled.

He was a therapist of the gentle school, person-centered by training and by temperament, and a colleague had dragged him to an ISTDP evening with the promise that it would at least be interesting. Ozias had read the reputation. Confrontational. Relentless. The therapy that yells at you until you cry, someone in his consultation group had called it, and everyone had laughed knowingly, and none of them had ever actually watched a session.

On screen, a therapist sat with a woman who had spent four sessions describing her husband in a voice like wet cardboard. "You say you want your marriage back," the therapist said, quietly. "And every time a real feeling about him rises, you go flat, like this, like now. I am not willing to sit here and watch you disappear for another month. Are you? Is this flat woman who you want to be with him?"

Ozias waited for the client to shatter. Instead she sat up. Actually sat up, color arriving in her face, and said with the first energy she had shown, "No. God, no, I hate this flatness." And the therapist smiled and said, "Good. Then let's not do the flatness. What is under it?"

Ozias unfolded his arms. Whatever he had just watched, it was not what the rumor had described. It had been, he admitted later, one of the more respectful things he had ever seen a therapist do: a refusal to abandon someone to their own avoidance.

This chapter takes the reputation head-on. You will learn what pressure and challenge actually mean in this model, why they only work inside an alliance, what the famous head-on collision is, how the field has genuinely changed since the early tapes, and where the line sits for you as an untrained reader. This is the chapter to read twice if ISTDP's intensity is what has kept you at arm's length.

8.1 What Pressure Actually Is

Pressure, in ISTDP, is sustained invitation toward feeling. That is the whole definition, and every word matters. Invitation: toward the client's own experience, not toward the therapist's agenda. Sustained: the invitation does not withdraw when the first defense arrives, or the fifth. Toward feeling: the destination is always the client's avoided inner life, never their submission.

In the room, pressure mostly sounds mundane. What do you feel toward her? Can we stay with that? Your mind wants to explain him; what does your body feel about him? Notice how quickly we left your father just now; shall we go back? Any single one of these questions is unremarkable. Pressure is what happens when a therapist asks them and then, warmly and without punishment, declines to be deflected, question after question, session after session. The intensity of ISTDP is not volume. It is consistency (Frederickson, 2013).

Why would consistency alone be so powerful? Because of what the client's system does in response. Remember the machinery: rising feeling triggers anxiety, anxiety summons defense. Steady pressure toward feeling means the defenses must keep working, visibly, in front of a witness who keeps kindly pointing at them. As resistance rises, something else rises with it, the compound Davanloo called complex transference feelings: irritation at this person who will not be managed, fear, guilt, and underneath, gathering force, the original buried feelings themselves, now stirring toward the surface (Davanloo, 1990). Pressure does not put feelings into anyone. It stops the removal system long enough for what was always there to arrive.

And the crucial calibration, which you can now appreciate because of Chapter 5.0: pressure is applied only as far as the body's channels say the system can bear. The therapist presses toward feeling while reading anxiety continuously, easing whenever the discharge leaves the striated channel (ten Have-de Labije & Neborsky, 2012). Pressure without that reading is not ISTDP. It is malpractice with ISTDP's vocabulary.

8.2 The Alliance Makes It Possible

Here is the part the rumor always omits: none of this is done to the client. It is done with them, under an agreement they made, in service of a goal they named.

Go back to Carwen and Ledger in section 7.4. Before any real pressure, an explicit contract: this is what you want changed, this is what changing it will require, do you want that from me. When Carwen later refuses Ledger's shrug, she is not overpowering him. She is keeping a promise he extracted from her. The model's writers are emphatic that the therapist allies with the client's healthy will against the client's defenses, never with the therapist's will against the client (Frederickson, 2013). The distinction is everything. It is the difference between a personal trainer you hired and a stranger shouting at you in a gym.

Something even stranger happens on the tapes, and Davanloo documented it repeatedly: as the therapist blocks defense after defense, most clients do not experience mounting persecution. They experience mounting respect, and something like hope, because a lifetime of successfully fending people off has finally met someone who cares enough not to be fended. Davanloo called the deep cooperation that rises the unconscious therapeutic alliance: beneath the surface struggle, the buried healthy part of the person starts actively helping, offering memories, dreams, and feelings toward the work (Davanloo, 1990). Clients say things afterward like: you were the first person who did not let me get away with it. That sentence, which sounds like a complaint, is spoken as gratitude.

You might be thinking this could still be rationalized coercion in gentler packaging. Keep that suspicion; it is healthy. The test is falsifiable and behavioral: in well-conducted ISTDP, the client can always disagree, redirect, or stop, the therapist tracks consent openly, and pressure eases the moment the body signals overload. Coercion overrides signals. This method is built out of reading them.

8.3 Example

The same intervention, done twice, so you can see exactly where the line runs.

Meet Bep, 55, who sought therapy after her adult son cut off contact. In her fourth session, describing his last message, her eyes filled, and instantly she reached for her oldest tool: "But you know, children these days, they need their space, I read an article about it."

Version one, pressure done badly. The therapist, hungry for the feeling he glimpsed, hardens: "There you go again with the articles. You always do this. You are avoiding, and until you stop avoiding, you will never get anywhere." Look at the anatomy of the failure. The defense has been framed as a character verdict, you always, delivered with the therapist's frustration riding on it, and the invitation has curdled into an accusation with no doorway back to the feeling. Bep apologizes, feels ashamed, and performs sadness for the rest of the session to appease him. Everything after this moment is compliance, which changes nothing.

Version two, pressure done well. The therapist leans in slightly, voice warm: "Can we notice something together? Tears came, just then, real ones, and within one breath the article arrived to take their place. That article has probably rescued you a thousand times. But your tears about your son are precisely what we are here for, and I do not want the article to take this from you too. Can we let the tears have their turn?" Same defense identified, same refusal to let it pass. But the defense is an action with a history, not a character flaw; the therapist's frustration is nowhere in the room; and the invitation back to feeling is standing wide open.

Bep, in the second version, cried for a long time, and what came with the tears surprised them both: not only grief but fury at her son, which she had been guarding even more closely than the sadness, because what kind of mother rages at the child she misses. That question, spoken aloud at last, became the therapy's real work.

What this means for you: pressure and attack can contain identical words about the defense. What separates them is frame, tone, ownership of frustration, and the open door back to feeling. Clients can tell the difference in their bones.

8.4 Collisions and How the Field Softened

Two more pieces complete the picture: the model's most famous maneuver, and its history of getting gentler.

At the far end of the intervention spectrum sits the **head-on collision**, a deliberate, structured confrontation with the client's entire resistance at once. The therapist lays out, sometimes at length, the full situation: here is what you came for, here is the wall you have built against it, here is what the wall will cost you if it wins, and here is the fact that I cannot want your life more than you do. It is reserved for high-resistance clients whose defenses are strangling the therapy, it requires precise psychodiagnosis and an established alliance, and in skilled hands it can be the moment the client's healthy will finally turns and fights for itself (Davanloo, 1990). You are reading a description, not an instruction. This intervention sits squarely on the far side of the line drawn in section 8.6.

Now the history, told honestly because you will encounter the old tapes and the old reputation. Early Davanloo-era work, filmed in the 1970s and 80s, can be startling to modern eyes: rapid, relentless, occasionally abrasive by today's norms. Some of that reflected the era's clinical culture, and some reflected a genuine limitation that the field's own development corrected. Later generations of ISTDP teachers, including the ones who built the graded approach for fragile clients, moved the model decisively toward calibration: matching intervention to capacity, attending explicitly to anxiety regulation, and framing the whole enterprise around the alliance (ten Have-de Labije & Neborsky, 2012). Contemporary texts foreground collaboration and warmth to a degree that surprises people who know only the rumor (Lied, 2025). The intensity was never the point. It was a means, and where gentler means serve better, the modern field uses them.

The fair summary: the reputation is not invented, it is outdated. Judge the model by its current best practice, the way you would want your own field judged.

8.5 Example

Bintou, whom you met in Chapter 5.0, can tell you what well-calibrated pressure feels like from the inside, because she described it to her therapist in their final session, and her description is worth more than a page of theory.

"For the first month," she said, "I kept waiting for you to be satisfied with my answers, like every other therapist was. You never were. You were kind about it, but you never once took the polite answer. And I want you to know I hated it for about three sessions." Her therapist laughed and asked what changed. Bintou thought about it. "I realized nobody had ever taken me that seriously. Everyone in my life accepts my fine-thanks. My husband accepts it. My doctor accepts it. You were the first person who acted like what was actually inside me mattered enough to keep asking. It felt like pressure, and then one day I noticed it felt like being valued."

She was quiet for a moment and then added the caveat that keeps this from being a commercial: "There were two sessions where it was too much and I told you so. And you stopped, both times. I think that is why I could trust the rest of it."

There is the entire chapter in a client's own words. Sustained invitation, experienced first as discomfort, then as respect. And underneath it, load-bearing, the two moments where she said too much and the pressure yielded immediately. The yielding is not a footnote to the method. It is the proof, delivered in the client's body, that the pressure was always invitation.

What this means for you: if you eventually train, your clients will run this same arc, hating it briefly, then trusting it. Both halves are normal. The yielding, when asked for, is what makes the second half possible.

8.6 When It Doesn't Work

The dangerous failure mode for readers of this chapter is not misunderstanding. It is enthusiasm. You finish these pages, the logic lands, and next Tuesday a client reaches for their favorite defense and you hear yourself say, "I am not willing to let you disappear." It sounded magnificent when the therapist on the tape said it.

Here is why that impulse must wait. The therapist on the tape was reading three anxiety channels in real time, held an explicit alliance contract, knew this client's capacity from careful psychodiagnosis, and had supervised training in what to do next, because the hardest part of pressure is not applying it, it is handling what rises when it works. You currently have none of those instruments. Pressure without them is a firework in a room you have not checked for gas.

Three things you can do instead, safely, starting now. First, practice not rescuing: when a client sits in productive discomfort, count five slow breaths before you speak. Most beginners rescue reflexively; unlearning that is real pressure training. Second, practice one honest noticing per session: "I notice we moved away from your mother just as tears came." Observation, offered once, without insistence. Third, keep watching the channels, because that skill is the foundation everything else stands on.

If a part of you is disappointed by these restraints, respect that part. It is the same healthy hunger that will eventually make training worthwhile. Chapter 12.0 will show you where to feed it properly.

8.7 One More Look

Pressure is sustained invitation toward feeling, and its intensity lives in consistency, not volume. It works only inside an explicit alliance, as a promise kept to the client's own stated will, and it is calibrated moment to moment against the body's anxiety channels, easing the instant the system signals overload. What rises under steady pressure, the mixture Davanloo called complex transference feelings, carries the buried past up with it, and beneath the surface struggle a deeper cooperation forms, the unconscious therapeutic alliance, the client's healthy side joining the work.

The head-on collision exists, at the far end of the spectrum, for trained hands only. The old tapes and the old reputation are real and outdated; the modern field runs on calibration and warmth. And for you, today, the line is bright: notice aloud, once, gently. Sustained pressure waits for training, and the part of you that finds that frustrating is the part worth training.

Chapter 9.0: Working With Fragile Clients

Hemi's previous therapist had meant well, and that was the problem.

Hemi was 31 and had arrived in that therapy carrying a childhood that social workers describe with the word chaotic and survivors describe with no word at all. The therapist, trained in an emotion-focused approach and genuinely kind, had done what her training suggested: invited Hemi toward his anger at his stepfather. What happened next frightened them both. Hemi's vision tunneled, the room went unreal, and he surfaced twenty minutes later in a parking lot with no memory of leaving the building.

He told his next therapist this story as a warning, the way you might tell a new mechanic about the last one who flooded the engine. The new therapist, ISTDP trained, heard it differently than Hemi expected. "Thank you," she said. "You have just told me exactly how we need to work. Your system protects you from big feeling by cutting the power. So we are not going to charge at big feeling. We are going to build, slowly, your capacity to have feelings with the power staying on. Small doses. You watching the dials with me. Nothing sudden."

Hemi, who had braced for either another charge or a polite referral elsewhere, felt something unfamiliar. Somebody had a plan that included his brakes, not just his accelerator.

This chapter is about the version of ISTDP built for people like Hemi, and it may be the most important chapter in the book for correcting the model's reputation. You will learn what fragility means here, how the graded format works, the red flags that tell a therapist to shift gears, and why the field's own writers regard this adaptation as some of its most valuable work.

9.1 What Fragile Means Here

In everyday speech, fragile sounds like an insult, so let's give it the precise, respectful meaning it carries in this model.

Fragility, in ISTDP terms, describes a nervous system whose anxiety, when feeling rises, does not discharge into the striated muscles, the green-light channel from Chapter 5.0, but instead goes quickly to the second and third channels: the gut, the fog, the fragmenting attention, the unreal room (ten Have-de Labije & Neborsky, 2012). It also describes a defensive system that, under load, reaches for the heavy machinery: dissociation, splitting, projection, the defenses that distort experience itself rather than merely redirecting it.

Notice what this definition is not. It is not a statement about weakness of character, intelligence, or worth. It is a statement about capacity, the amount of rising feeling a system can currently contain while keeping thinking and perception online. Capacity is not fixed. It is built, which is the entire premise of this chapter.

Where does low capacity come from? Broadly, from histories where overwhelming feeling arrived early and often, with no adult helping to contain it. A child's capacity develops through thousands of repetitions of feeling-with-help. Where help never came, or where the helpers were the danger, the system learned emergency measures instead: cut the power, leave the body, split the world into simple pieces. As always in this model, the pathology was once protection (Frederickson, 2013).

Roughly speaking, you will hear the field sort clients along a spectrum of resistance and fragility. On one side, high-resistance clients like Ledger: solid capacity, armored defenses, systems that can take robust pressure. On the other, fragile clients like Hemi, where the standard approach is not just unhelpful but contraindicated. Reading which client is in front of you is precisely the psychodiagnosis of Chapter 7.0, and it is the first thing the first session must establish.

9.2 The Graded Format

The adaptation built for fragility is called the **graded format**, and its logic fits in one sentence: instead of pressing feeling upward until it breaks through, you raise feeling a small amount, stop, regulate, help the client observe what just happened, and repeat, building capacity like a muscle across many gentle repetitions (Abbass, 2015).

Watch the shape of one graded cycle, because the shape is the method. The therapist invites a small rise of feeling: not what do you feel about your entire stepfather, but staying just with that one memory of the kitchen doorway, what starts to happen in your body. The moment anxiety shows the first sign of leaving the striated channel, a hint of stomach, the earliest wisp of fog, the therapist stops the rise and shifts to regulation: naming what is happening, bringing attention to concrete bodily detail, engaging the client's thinking. Then, and this step is the secret engine, they recap together: did you notice, feeling rose, your anxiety went to your stomach, we paused, it settled. The client is not just having an experience; they are learning, consciously, how their own system works, and every observed cycle expands what the system can hold next time (ten Have-de Labije & Neborsky, 2012).

If Chapter 8.0 was an expedition, this is physiotherapy: unglamorous, repetitive, incremental, and cumulative in a way that startles people. Months of small cycles produce clients who can feel real anger, real grief, with thinking intact, often for the first time in their lives. The buried feelings do eventually get their full experience, as in any ISTDP. The road is longer, and it is the same destination.

One reframe for you as a reader: the graded format is not ISTDP with the good parts removed. The field's own literature treats capacity-building with fragile clients as among the model's most sophisticated achievements, demanding more precision from the therapist, not less (Frederickson, 2013). Gentleness, done this deliberately, is advanced technique.

9.3 Example

Watch a single graded session, close up.

Louka, 27, worked in a supermarket warehouse and had been referred after a string of panic attacks and a hospital admission for chest pain with clean cardiology results. His first session revealed the pattern: any question that stirred feeling sent his anxiety straight to the second channel, chest tight, stomach lurching, and beyond it, quickly, toward the third, thoughts scattering like startled birds.

Session eleven. His therapist asks about his sister's wedding, where Louka was seated away from the family table. A flicker crosses his face. "What just stirred, right then?" the therapist asks. Louka: "I do not know. Something." Therapist: "Where in your body?" Louka: "Chest. Like a fist." Therapist, watching him carefully: "Let's stay just at the edge of the fist. Not into it. If it is a feeling toward someone, who would it point at?" Louka: "My mother. She arranged the seating." His hands, unnoticed by him, have curled into fists on his knees. Striated. The system is holding.

Then his breathing shallows and he says the room feels a bit far away. First wisp of the third channel. The therapist stops instantly, without alarm: "Good, pause there. Look at me. Feel your feet on the floor. Your body just did the thing we know it does. Describe the far-away, in plain words." They spend three minutes on plain words. The room returns. And then the recap: "Did you catch the whole arc? Anger toward your mother started to rise, your hands made fists, which is new and healthy, then your system pulled the fog lever, we paused, and you came back in three minutes. A year ago that would have been a panic attack in a parking lot. That is capacity, being built, in real time."

Louka looked at his own hands, still half-curled, with something like wonder. Progress made visible is fuel, and graded work runs on it.

What this means for you: notice that in ten minutes of session, the feeling itself advanced perhaps one degree. The capacity advanced more. In graded work, that exchange rate is not a compromise. It is the treatment.

9.4 Red Flags and Gear Changes

How does a therapist know, in the moment, that the standard road is wrong and the graded road is needed? The model gives concrete answers, and even as an untrained reader you should know them, because they are the safety rails around everything this book has described.

The signals for shifting to the graded approach include: anxiety that moves to the smooth muscle channel or toward cognitive-perceptual disruption at low levels of rising feeling; any appearance of dissociation, the fog, the unreal room, the lost minutes; heavy reliance on reality-distorting defenses like projection, where disowned feeling is experienced as coming from other people, including the therapist; histories that predict low capacity, including severe early trauma and previous flooding experiences in therapy like Hemi's; and active conditions, from psychotic vulnerability to acute crisis, where any uncovering work needs extreme care or a different treatment entirely (Abbass, 2015).

Notice that most of these are exactly the third-channel and heavy-machinery signs from Chapters 5.0 and 6.0. The skills stack: the anxiety channels you learned to watch are the same instruments that route each client to the right road.

Two honest additions. First, capacity is not a fixed label a client wears; the same person can need graded work in a crisis season and tolerate standard work a year later, so the reading never stops. Second, and this matters for your professional humility: sometimes the reading says this client needs something other than me. A trained ISTDP therapist who identifies needs beyond their competence refers onward, and that judgment is considered part of the method, not a failure of it. Short-term dynamic therapy has evidence across a wide range of conditions, including somatic and treatment-resistant presentations (Abbass, Town, & Driessen, 2012), and no therapy is for everyone, a fact the Cochrane reviewers make quietly clear across their careful tables (Abbass et al., 2014).

9.5 Example

The referral judgment deserves its own story, because beginners imagine expertise as never being out of your depth, and expertise is actually knowing the depth precisely.

Auguste had been practicing ISTDP for four years when a new client arrived: 44, recently discharged from an inpatient unit, with a dissociative disorder diagnosis, an eating disorder history, and a childhood that made Auguste's notes hard to write. The client was motivated, articulate, and desperate for exactly the kind of deep emotional work ISTDP promises.

Auguste ran two careful assessment sessions and watched the instruments. Fog arrived at the mildest emotional questions. Time went strange for the client twice in one hour. Between sessions, a voicemail arrived at 2 a.m. that suggested the alliance was already carrying more weight than it could bear. Auguste took the recordings to supervision and said, out loud, the sentence that four years earlier would have felt like failure: "I think this person needs more than I can safely provide."

The supervisor agreed. Together they arranged a referral to a specialized trauma service with psychiatric support, and Auguste handled the handover with the same care as any intervention, naming it honestly to the client: not a rejection, but a matching of need to resource. The client was hurt anyway, and said so, and Auguste sat with that without retracting the decision. Months later, word came back through the service that the client had stabilized and begun structured trauma work.

It is not a triumphant story. It is a correct one, and the difference between those two things is roughly the difference between a beginner and a professional.

What this means for you: the graded format extends ISTDP's reach remarkably far, and it does not extend it infinitely. Knowing the edge of your competence, and acting on it kindly, is a clinical skill of the same rank as any in this book.

9.6 When It Doesn't Work

Here is the failure this chapter predictably produces in readers who are practicing clinicians: diagnostic vertigo. You will meet a client next week, spot one sigh and one foggy moment, and spiral about which road they need, standard or graded, robust or fragile, and feel like a fraud for not knowing.

You cannot know yet, and you are not supposed to. Formal psychodiagnosis, the confident routing of a client onto the right road, is a trained skill built on hundreds of supervised observations. What you have after one book chapter is a vocabulary, and a vocabulary is not a license. The vertigo is the feeling of taking the vocabulary seriously, which is to your credit.

Three things to do with it. First, use the vocabulary descriptively, never prescriptively: in your notes, record what you actually saw, sighed four times, went vague when father mentioned, reported stomach knot, without leaping to route the client anywhere.

Second, hold one question gently across your caseload: whose anxiety seems to skip the muscles? Those are the clients about whom you should be most conservative with any emotionally evocative technique, from any model you practice. Third, if you supervise or refer, start including capacity language in those conversations; you will be surprised how much it clarifies.

And permission: if a client in front of you is fogging, dissociating, or somatically flooding, you do not need this book's model to know what to do. Slow down, ground them, stay warm, and consult. That was good practice before ISTDP named the channels, and it is good practice now.

9.7 Where You Are Now

Fragility, in this model, is a precise and respectful word: a nervous system whose anxiety abandons the muscles early, heading for the gut and the fog, and whose defenses reach for heavy machinery like dissociation. It signals limited capacity, and capacity is buildable, which is the graded format's entire premise: raise feeling a little, stop, regulate, observe the cycle together, repeat, physiotherapy for the emotional system.

The red flags that route a client to the graded road are the same third-channel signs you learned in Chapter 5.0, plus reality-distorting defenses and histories that predict flooding. The reading never stops, capacity changes across seasons of a life, and sometimes the right reading is a referral, made kindly and without shame.

Hold this chapter against the rumor from Chapter 8.0 and notice what you now know: the model famous for intensity contains, at its most sophisticated, some of the gentlest, most patient technique in the therapy world. Both are true, because both are calibration.

Chapter 10.0: Breakthroughs and What Follows

The moment, when it finally came for Kylara, did not look like the movies.

She was 36, fourteen sessions in, and the work that day had circled her grandmother, the one adult of her childhood who had been safe, and who had died the spring Kylara turned eleven, after which nobody in the household ever mentioned her again. Kylara had learned the family curriculum perfectly: feelings are private weather, and grief is self-indulgence.

Her therapist had spent the session doing what you now know how to watch: steady invitation toward feeling, defenses noticed kindly, sighs deepening, hands working. And then Kylara stopped mid-sentence, and her face did something that her therapist later described as the look of a person hearing their name called from a very long way off. "She used to sing while she peeled apples," Kylara said, in a voice that belonged to someone eleven years old, and then the grief arrived, all of it, twenty-five years of it, in waves that bent her forward in the chair.

Here is what the movies get wrong. The therapist did not lean back, satisfied, as the credits rolled. The most important work of the session was just beginning. Because after the wave passed, and it did pass, Kylara sat up into a strange, washed clarity, and memories were arriving in vivid specific color, and what she and her therapist did with the next twenty minutes would determine what this moment became: a strange intense Tuesday, or a turning point.

This chapter is about breakthroughs: what actually happens in them, what rises with them, and why the unglamorous work that follows, consolidation, is where the change is actually made. It also tells you honestly what the research says, and what happens for the many clients whose change never includes a scene like Kylara's at all.

10.1 What a Breakthrough Actually Is

The field's term for moments like Kylara's is the **breakthrough of complex feelings into conscious experience**, or in Davanloo's stronger phrase, unlocking the unconscious, and the definition matters: it is the direct, bodily experience of previously buried feeling, not a realization about it (Davanloo, 1990).

The distinction is everything, and you have been building toward it all book. Orson, back in Chapter 1.0, had realizations about his mother for decades; his castle tour was made of them. A breakthrough is categorically different: the feeling itself, arriving in the body at full strength, with the defenses that always intercepted it standing aside. Grief that bends you forward. Rage that arrives with heat and impulse. Love and longing with a force that embarrasses the adult feeling them. The person is not thinking about the feeling. They are, at last, having it.

Two signatures distinguish genuine breakthroughs on the tapes, and both appeared in Kylara's session. First, the feeling is somatically complete: it moves through the body with direction and energy, and then it genuinely passes, leaving not depletion but a distinctive calm the literature keeps reaching for words like clarity and lightness to describe (Coughlin Della Selva, 2004). Second, and this is the eerie, reliable part Davanloo filmed over and over: the breakthrough unlocks memory. As the feeling completes, specific vivid memories surface, often ones the person had not consciously held for decades, the apple-peeling, the exact kitchen, the song. The buried feeling and the buried history were filed together, and they come up together (Davanloo, 1990).

One honest note before we go further: a breakthrough is not an exorcism. Nothing leaves the person. What changes is that a feeling which could not be experienced now has been, which means the machinery built to prevent it has, at least once, proven unnecessary. Once is not transformation. Once is a door, standing open.

10.2 The Grief Under the Rage

Here is the pattern that surprises every newcomer to the tapes, and it deserves its own section because it will reorganize how you think about anger.

In case after filmed case, when the most defended feeling finally breaks through, it comes in layers, and the layers run in a sequence. First, typically, rage, often murderous in its imagery, toward the loved person who caused the early pain. The client experiences the rage somatically, sometimes in a guided fantasy of what the impulse wants to do, which is the part of ISTDP that sounds most alarming secondhand and, on tape, is most obviously liberating firsthand. But the rage is almost never the bottom. As it completes, guilt rises about the rage, because the rage is aimed at someone the person also loved. And under the guilt, at the bottom of everything, is grief and love: sorrow for the relationship as it actually was, longing for the relationship it should have been (Malan & Coughlin Della Selva, 2006).

Rage, guilt, grief, love. The sequence explains something that puzzles beginners: why a therapy so associated with anger produces endings so full of tenderness. The anger was never the destination. It was the crust, and the model presses through it because what is underneath, the guilt-soaked love, is what actually binds the symptoms. In the theory's terms, it is largely the unconscious guilt about rage toward loved ones that drives self-punishment: the self-attack, the sabotaged successes, the depressions that arrive precisely when life goes well (Frederickson, 2013).

You might be thinking this sounds too tidy, too archaeological, layers in a prescribed order. Fair, and hold the skepticism. Real sessions are messier, layers interleave and return, and not every client's material follows the diagram. But the broad sequence recurs on enough independent tape, across enough therapists, that the field treats it as a reliable map of defended feeling toward loved-and-hurtful figures, which describes most of the figures that matter.

10.3 Example

Let's stay with Kylara, because what happened after her wave of grief is the part beginners skip and professionals study.

Her therapist did not rush in. The wave passed, and Kylara sat quietly, and the therapist let the quiet be. Then, gently: "What is happening now, inside?" Kylara, still in that washed voice: "It is quiet in there. I do not remember it ever being quiet in there." More memories were surfacing, unforced: her grandmother's kitchen, the smell of it, and a specific afternoon of being sung to while feverish. And then something else surfaced with them: "I am so angry at my mother. She threw out Nana's things while I was at school. I came home and the room was empty. I had forgotten that. How do you forget a thing like that?"

Watch what the therapist does with the remaining minutes, because this is **consolidation** beginning: the work of connecting the felt experience to the pattern of a whole life. Together, unhurried, they traced it: the grief that was forbidden, the anger at her mother that was doubly forbidden, and the machinery an eleven-year-old built to contain both, which was the same machinery, twenty-five years later, that made Kylara the colleague who organized everyone's leaving parties and wept at no funerals, the partner whose warmth had what her husband called a sealed lid. The empty room and the sealed lid were the same room. She saw it, not as an interpretation delivered from across the room, but as a fact of her own biography, felt from the inside.

Sessions fifteen through twenty were consolidation almost entirely: the lid loosening in specific current relationships, backslides examined without alarm, the new capacity tested against the living family. Her mother, for the record, did not change at all. Kylara grieved that too, which is what consolidation is for.

What this means for you: the breakthrough opened the door; the walking through it was cognitive, relational, and slow. Feeling without integration is an event. Feeling with integration is change.

10.4 What the Research Says

Time to put numbers where the drama has been, because a model this vivid needs its claims checked.

The central empirical question is not just does ISTDP help, Chapter 1.0 covered that, but does the breakthrough itself matter? The model stakes everything on those moments; a skeptic could reply that clients improve for ordinary reasons, alliance and attention, and the fireworks are decoration. The Halifax group tested this directly in a real-world tertiary service: across a large treated sample, clients improved substantially, and clients whose therapies included unlockings, the breakthrough experiences, showed greater symptom reduction than those whose therapies did not (Johansson, Town, & Abbass, 2014). Correlational, not proof of mechanism, the authors are careful, and it is exactly what the model predicts.

Around that sit the outcome findings you already know: meta-analytic support for ISTDP across conditions including treatment-resistant ones (Abbass, Town, & Driessen, 2012), and randomized evidence in genuinely hard populations, including a controlled trial for treatment-resistant depression, where ISTDP outperformed usual care by a moderate to large margin and produced far higher remission rates (Town et al., 2017), an advantage still present at eighteen-month follow-up (Town et al., 2020). Follow-up patterns across the family of dynamic therapies suggest gains that hold or grow after termination, consistent with the idea that something structural, not just symptomatic, has shifted (Shedler, 2010).

The honest limits, stated plainly because you deserve them: samples in ISTDP-specific studies are often modest, many researchers are also proponents, replication by fully independent groups remains thinner than anyone would like, and unlocking is defined and rated within the model's own framework. Promising, coherent, and still earning its way. If a colleague tells you the breakthrough research is airtight, or that it is nothing, they are both overclaiming.

10.5 Example

Now the corrective story, because Kylara's arc, left alone, would teach you something false.

Firdous, 52, whom Sama lost in Chapter 7.0, eventually found her way to a different therapist, one who read her capacity correctly and took the graded road. Two years of it. And here is the thing: in two years of genuinely successful therapy, Firdous never had a Kylara moment. No wave, no unlocked kitchen, no cinematic bend in the chair.

What she had instead was increments. The panic attacks spaced out, then largely stopped. She noticed anger at her late husband's family within days instead of never. She held her daughter's criticism without a week of stomach trouble. In session sixty-something, describing her redundancy, the one that had originally brought her to therapy, she cried, ordinary quiet tears, and did not apologize for them, and later told her therapist that not apologizing had felt like the biggest thing she had ever done in a chair.

Was Firdous's therapy a lesser ISTDP? The field's own answer is no. In graded work, the breakthrough is often distributed: a hundred small completions of feeling instead of one large one, capacity accreting until the person's life is different, with no single scene to point at (Abbass, 2015). The dramatic unlockings cluster in higher-capacity, high-resistance treatments; they are one shape of success, not its definition. Firdous's outcome, measured in the mornings of her actual life, matched anything in this chapter.

She did once ask her therapist, having read something online, why she never had the big cathartic thing. Her therapist said: "You have been having it. In installments. You just kept mistaking it for Tuesday." Firdous liked that enough to repeat it to her daughter.

What this means for you: hold the movie version loosely. Some change arrives as a wave, some as a tide, and a therapist who only values waves will miss, and undervalue, most of the actual healing in front of them.

10.6 When It Doesn't Work

The predictable distortion this chapter creates is breakthrough hunger. Readers, and young therapists especially, fall in love with the wave: they start measuring sessions, their clients', eventually their own therapy, against the cinematic standard, and quietly grading everything gentler as failure.

Why it happens: the breakthrough is the most narratable thing in psychotherapy. Stories need scenes, and Kylara's kitchen is a scene, and Firdous's sixty increments are not. Your memory will keep the scene and discard the tide, and then your expectations will follow your memory.

Three correctives. First, whenever you recall Kylara, deliberately recall Firdous in the same breath; pair them permanently, the wave and the tide. Second, if you are a practicing clinician, audit one long-term client for distributed change: list five small feelings they now complete that they could not at intake. That list is breakthrough material, in installments. Third, notice any impulse to provoke big affect in your current work, from any model, and treat the impulse itself as the thing to examine, ideally in supervision. Wanting the scene is about the therapist. The client only needs the change.

And if you find the whole topic sits strangely with you, too intense, too theatrical, park it. Chapters 11.0 and 12.0 do not depend on your loving this one, and plenty of working ISTDP therapists came around to breakthroughs slowly, from exactly your seat.

10.7 Closing Thoughts

A breakthrough is the direct bodily experience of a feeling that was buried, not an insight about it, and on the tapes it carries two signatures: the feeling completes somatically, leaving a distinctive calm, and it unlocks memory, the buried history surfacing with the buried feeling. Defended feeling toward loved figures tends to arrive in layers, rage first, then guilt, then the grief and love underneath, which is why a therapy famous for anger ends so often in tenderness, and why the model ties self-punishing symptoms to unconscious guilt about rage at people we loved.

The moment itself is a door, not the change. Consolidation, connecting the felt experience to the pattern of a life and testing the new capacity against living relationships, is where the door gets walked through. The research offers real support, improvement linked to unlocking, randomized evidence in hard populations, alongside real limits worth stating.

And some of the best outcomes never contain a scene at all. The wave and the tide. Keep both, permanently, and you will be a fairer judge of change than most of the field.

Chapter 11.0: ISTDP Next to Other Therapies

Emjay ran a CBT practice, a good one, and had a client she privately called the Teflon man.

He was cooperative, intelligent, and completely unchanged by fourteen sessions of skilled cognitive work. He completed thought records like a star pupil. He could restructure a cognition in his sleep. And his depression sat exactly where it had been in session one, because, Emjay slowly realized, the worksheets never touched him. He handled them the way he handled everything: from behind glass.

She brought the case to a consultation group, where a colleague who had done ISTDP core training asked an odd question: "When he talks about his father, what does his body do?" Emjay had no idea. She had never watched. The next session, she watched. When his father came up, the Teflon man's jaw tightened, one long sigh escaped, and then he made a small joke and asked about homework. Glass, it turned out, had a manufacturing process, and it ran right there in the room, between the worksheets.

Emjay did not throw away her CBT. What happened instead is the subject of this chapter: she learned where her model ended and what the therapy next door knew about the territory beyond it. This chapter puts ISTDP beside the approaches you are most likely to know already, CBT and its relatives, the experiential dynamic cousins like AEDP and EFT, and traditional long-term psychodynamic therapy, so you can see clearly what is shared, what is genuinely different, what you can borrow tomorrow, and how to think about fit, including the possibility that this model is not your fit at all.

11.1 Next to CBT

Start with the comparison most readers carry in the door, because most working therapists today grew up professionally inside cognitive-behavioral thinking.

The core difference is the theory of where suffering lives. CBT locates it, broadly, in the content of cognition: distorted thoughts and beliefs generate painful feelings and unhelpful behavior, so you change the thoughts and behavior. ISTDP locates suffering in the avoidance of feeling: buried emotion generates anxiety and defenses, and the defenses generate symptoms, so you help the person experience what they have been avoiding. To a CBT therapist, Thibault's "I am worthless" from Chapter 3.0 is a distortion to be examined against evidence. To an ISTDP therapist, it is a defense in motion, and the working question is what feeling just went underground (Frederickson, 2013).

Both models are honest, structured, and results-oriented, which is why clinicians move between them more easily than the rhetoric suggests. And the border is genuinely busier than it used to be. On the CBT side, the field has moved steadily toward emotion and experience: exposure has always worked by having the feared experience rather than debating it, acceptance and commitment therapy explicitly targets experiential avoidance, the refusal to have inner experience, as a core pathology (Hayes, Strosahl, & Wilson, 2011), and the transdiagnostic Unified Protocol trains clients to approach, tolerate, and stay with emotion (Barlow et al., 2017). Read those sentences again and notice something: the therapy families are converging on the same enemy, avoidance, from different directions.

What ISTDP adds that a CBT-trained reader will feel immediately: the moment-to-moment reading of the body's anxiety channels, the systematic, compassionate confrontation of defenses as they operate live, and the use of the therapy relationship itself as the primary arena. Emjay's Teflon man had never been asked what he felt toward her about doing all this homework. When she finally asked, watching his jaw, the glass got its first crack.

11.2 The Experiential Cousins

Now the family comparisons, which matter because these are the therapies most often shortlisted alongside ISTDP by the same curious clinicians.

AEDP, accelerated experiential dynamic psychotherapy, is the closest relative, founded by Diana Fosha out of the same lineage. It shares the conviction that the direct experience of previously avoided emotion heals, and it shares the attention to moment-to-moment process. The divergence is stance and emphasis. Where ISTDP works systematically against defenses, AEDP leads with the therapist's explicit warmth and affirmation, seeks to bypass defenses by making the relationship safe enough that they stand down, and gives unusual attention to positive affect: the felt experience of transformation itself, processed as it happens (Fosha, 2000). Caricaturing only slightly: ISTDP unlocks the door; AEDP warms the house until the door opens.

Emotion-focused therapy, from Leslie Greenberg's research tradition, arrives at a similar destination from humanistic and process-research roots: emotion is the master signal, clients are helped to access, deepen, and transform emotional states, often through structured tasks like chair work (Greenberg, 2015). EFT shares ISTDP's core wager, that emotional experience, not insight, drives change, and differs in its softer stance toward defenses and its origins outside the psychodynamic frame.

And classical long-term psychodynamic therapy is the ancestor at the table: same map of conflict, transference, and defense, radically different activity level and timeline. The honest way to say it: ISTDP is psychodynamic theory driven at experiential speed, and it was built, as Chapter 2.0 told you, precisely out of impatience with the ancestor's pace.

Does the evidence crown one cousin? No, and be suspicious of anyone who says otherwise. The experiential dynamic family shows solid pooled efficacy across fifty-seven randomized trials (Lilliengren et al., 2025), dynamic therapy broadly performs comparably to other bona fide treatments (Shedler, 2010), and head-to-head trials between the cousins are rare. Fit, for a given client and a given therapist, remains the live question, which is where this chapter is headed.

11.3 Example

Watch what borrowing looks like when it is done with respect for both models.

Emjay, back with the Teflon man, did not attempt amateur ISTDP; Chapter 8.0 told you why, and she knew it too. What she did was integrate three things that required no pressure techniques at all. First, she started watching the body, and shared what she saw, in her own model's collaborative language: "I notice when your father comes up, your jaw tightens and then a joke arrives. I wonder if the joke is doing a job." Second, she began treating his relationship to the therapy itself as material: what was it like to hand in perfect homework to her, week after week? What would an imperfect week feel like? Third, she stopped accepting reports about feelings and started asking for the feelings themselves, in-session, in the body, and waiting.

The case turned, not cinematically but definitely. The Teflon man, invited past the joke one afternoon, said the first unrehearsed sentence of the treatment: "If I actually feel this stuff, I do not think it stops." There it was, the belief under the glass, and notice something delicious: it was a cognition, exactly the kind of catastrophic prediction CBT was built to test. Emjay, fluent in her own model, treated it as one, and they designed the gentlest possible behavioral experiment: feel one feeling, in session, with her, and measure what actually happens. The feeling was grief, it lasted four minutes, and it stopped. The Teflon man sat in the quiet afterward and said, "Huh," which in his dialect was a breakthrough.

Emjay kept her license plate firmly CBT. But her intake questions changed, her eyes changed, and two years later she enrolled in an ISTDP pre-core course, not to convert, but because she wanted the trained version of what she had been improvising.

What this means for you: the borrowable layer of ISTDP is observational and relational, watch the body, use the room, ask for the feeling itself, and it upgrades any model without impersonating this one.

11.4 The Question of Fit

The comparison that actually matters is not between therapies in the abstract. It is between a therapy and a particular human, and there are two humans in every dyad. Take the client first.

The honest sales pitch for ISTDP is strongest for the clients other approaches strand: the insight-rich and unchanged, like Orson; the somatizers whose bodies speak for them, like Keva, backed by the somatic evidence base (Abbass, Kisely, & Kroenke, 2009); the treatment-resistant, where randomized evidence exists (Town et al., 2017); and the armored competent, like Mehreen, whose defenses are excellent enough to defeat gentler methods. The model is a poorer first choice where capacity is very low and stabilization is the need of the hour, though Chapter 9.0 showed you how far the graded road extends, and it is simply unavailable, practically, where no trained practitioner exists within reach, which remains true of large parts of the world.

Now the therapist, meaning possibly you. Models are not just toolkits; they are temperamental homes. ISTDP asks its practitioners to be comfortable with high emotional voltage, to tolerate being the target of feeling, to watch themselves on video without dying of shame, and to sustain warm insistence where other trainings taught retreat. Some excellent therapists discover this fits like a glove they had always been missing. Others discover, honestly, that it grates against their grain, and that discovery is worth respecting.

A self-assessment, in four questions, no scoring, just notice your gut. When a client cries hard, is your first impulse to accompany or to soothe it away? When a client is angry at you, can you stay curious? Does the phrase watch yourself on video with a supervisor produce dread you could work with, or dread that answers the question? And when you watched the therapists in this book decline to accept the polite answer, did something in you lean in, or wince and keep wincing? Lean-in readers, Chapter 12.0 was written for you. Wince-and-keep-wincing readers, the next story is yours.

11.5 Example

Corby did everything right and chose differently, and this book would be dishonest without a story like theirs.

Corby was a therapist of six years' standing who read the introductory literature, watched the demonstration videos, attended a two-day ISTDP workshop, and even role-played the techniques in a practice triad, where something instructive happened: asked to maintain pressure on a colleague playing a resistant client, Corby physically could not. Not would not, could not; their voice kept softening the intervention into apology. The workshop leader, who was good, did not treat this as failure. She asked what Corby was feeling, and Corby, to their own surprise, said, "Like I am being cruel, and I know I am not, and the knowing does not help."

Corby sat with that for a month, honestly, the way this book has been asking you to sit with things. The conclusion was not that ISTDP was wrong, or that the workshop had misrepresented it;

Corby had seen with their own eyes that the pressure on the tapes was alliance-based and kind. The conclusion was about grain: Corby's clinical gifts, considerable ones, ran through patience, softness, and indirection, and a model requiring sustained insistence would have Corby practicing against their own temperament for years, which is expensive for the therapist and, ultimately, felt by clients.

Corby trained in emotion-focused therapy instead, where the same core wager, feeling over insight, is pursued through structured tasks rather than sustained pressure (Greenberg, 2015), and became, by all accounts including their own, a better therapist than before, partly because of everything the ISTDP detour had taught them about watching bodies and respecting avoidance. Two of Corby's referrals each year now go to a local ISTDP practitioner, sent knowledgeably, for exactly the armored clients that softness strands.

What this means for you: studying this model pays off even if you never practice it. And choosing a different home, from an informed position, is not a failure of nerve. It is psychodiagnosis, applied to yourself, and it is the same skill this whole book has been teaching.

11.6 When It Doesn't Work

The failure mode of comparison chapters is conversion fever, in either direction. Some readers finish and quietly decide their existing training is the problem with their careers, and begin dismissing tools that served their clients for years. Others feel their home model criticized, bristle, and dismiss everything here as psychodynamic marketing. Both are the same error: treating models as teams to join rather than lenses to hold.

Why it happens: professional identity is identity, and this chapter has been poking it. A new lens that explains your hardest cases is exhilarating in a way that feels like revelation, and threat to an old lens feels personal. Neither feeling is information about the models.

Three things to try. First, apply the one-case test: take your single most stuck client and write two paragraphs, one explaining the stuckness in your home model's terms, one in ISTDP's terms. Keep the pair; notice which paragraph suggests a next move. Second, borrow before you convert: run the three observational upgrades from section 11.3 for one month inside your existing model, and let results, not enthusiasm, tell you what they are worth. Third, if the fever persists, set a one-year rule: no training commitments to any new model until you have watched real full-length session recordings of it, not workshop highlights, because highlight reels convert everyone.

And permission, again, to end where Corby ended. This chapter's job was a fair comparison, not a recruitment. If your reading of it is a clearer commitment to the model you already practice, the chapter worked.

11.7 The Main Ideas

Set beside CBT, the deep difference is the address of suffering: distorted cognition versus avoided feeling, worksheets versus the machinery running between them, and yet the families are converging on avoidance as the shared enemy, with ACT and the Unified Protocol naming it outright. Set beside the cousins, AEDP warms where ISTDP works the defenses directly, EFT reaches similar experiential goals through structured tasks, and classical psychodynamic therapy is the same theory at a fraction of the speed. The evidence supports the family without crowning a cousin.

What travels tomorrow into any practice: watch the body, use the room, ask for the feeling itself. What does not travel without training: everything in Chapter 8.0.

And fit is bidirectional. Some clients need exactly this model; some therapists are built for it and some are honestly not, and finding out which you are, from an informed position, is a professional achievement either way. For the lean-in readers, one chapter remains, and it is the practical one: the door itself.

Chapter 12.0: Your Training Path

Zowie kept the email in her drafts folder for eleven days.

It was three sentences long, an inquiry about joining a pre-core ISTDP course, and she could not send it. Every time her cursor hovered, the same committee convened in her head. You are a counselor, not a psychiatrist; these people will be doctors. You have been qualified six years; they will ask why you waited. And the big one, the one with teeth: they film you. Everyone will watch you work, and then everyone will know.

What finally got the email sent was not courage. It was a sentence from a colleague who had trained years earlier and knew the committee well, because she had hosted her own version of it. "Zowie," she said, "the video is not there to expose you. It is there so you stop having to guess. You have been guessing alone in a room for six years. How is that gentler?"

Zowie sent the email. Three years later, she finished core training, having nearly quit once, in month four, for reasons this chapter will be honest about. She now says the training rebuilt her from the eyes down, and that she would not hand back a single one of the excruciating video reviews. Both halves of that sentence are true, and both halves are what this chapter owes you.

This is the practical chapter. What the training ladder actually looks like, rung by rung. What it costs, in money, time, and pride. How to vet a trainer. What to read, in what order. And what to do with the next ninety days if you finish this book and want to keep moving, including a self-study plan that costs almost nothing. No mystique, no gatekeeping, just the map.

12.1 The Ladder Itself

The ISTDP training path is unusually standardized across the world, which is good news: once you know the rungs, you can evaluate any provider against them.

The first rung is what you are doing right now: reading, plus watching. Books, recorded demonstrations, introductory webinars and workshops. Free to cheap, no prerequisites, and genuinely valuable; you have just spent eleven chapters on this rung, and section 12.4 will tell you what to read next.

The second rung is the **pre-core** course, sometimes called an introductory or preparatory course. Typically a series of workshop days spread over some months, mixing theory, video demonstration, and skills practice. This is where you discover, at modest cost, what Corby discovered in Chapter 11.0: how the model sits in your actual hands. Expect fees in the region of several hundred dollars or pounds; at the time of writing, published prices for a stand-alone two-day introduction sit in the low hundreds, with one UK provider advertising 450 pounds, and figures vary by provider, length, and country (ISTDP UK, n.d.). Check the current provider pages rather than trusting any number printed in a book, including this one.

The third rung is the big one: **core training**, the internationally standard format of which is three years, in a small closed group, commonly capped somewhere around a dozen trainees, meeting for multi-day blocks several times a year, combining theory, skill drills, and, centrally, supervised review of video from each trainee's real practice (ISTDP UK, n.d.). Core training normally requires that you are a licensed or registered mental health professional with an active caseload, because the training runs on your own recorded sessions. This is the rung where the model actually transfers from books into hands.

Beyond core lie advanced supervision, specialist workshops, and eventually, for some, teacher training under the umbrella of the International Experiential Dynamic Therapy Association, which maintains standards and a directory across countries (International Experiential Dynamic Therapy Association, n.d.). But the working summary is simple: read, then pre-core, then core, then supervised forever, which last part is only half a joke.

12.2 Costs Money Pride

Now the accounting nobody publishes in one place, delivered in the three currencies that actually get spent.

Money. Reading and watching: tens of dollars. Pre-core: several hundred, as above. Core training: budget for course fees across three years that commonly land, in total, in the several-thousands range depending on country and provider, plus travel to training blocks, plus the recording equipment and secure storage for session video, plus, realistically, some individual supervision between blocks. It is a serious professional investment, comparable to other advanced psychotherapy trainings, and it is spread across years, which is how most trainees survive it. If the number makes you wince, remember you are standing on rung one, which costs almost nothing, and rung two exists precisely so you can test commitment before the big spend.

Time. Pre-core: workshop days plus reading. Core: the blocks themselves, preparation of video and process notes before each block, and the slow-motion work of reviewing your own sessions between meetings. Trainees with full caseloads describe it as a steady background load rather than a crushing one, with spikes before each block.

Pride. Here is the honest currency, and the one that nearly took Zowie out in month four. Core training's engine is video review: you, your real client, your real fumbles, on a screen, in front of a supervisor and your group. The first reviews are, by near-universal testimony, mortifying. You will watch yourself miss signals this book taught you to name. You will hear your own voice soften a crucial intervention into mush, as Corby's did. And then, if the group is well led, something shifts: the exposure you feared becomes the fastest feedback loop you have ever worked inside, the thing research on therapist development keeps pointing toward, deliberate practice on your own actual performance rather than years of unexamined repetition (Rousmaniere, 2024). Guessing alone in a room, it turns out, was the harsher deal all along.

12.3 Example

Month four, the near-quitting, because Zowie insists this part be told.

Her first full video review fell in the second block of core training. She had chosen, deliberately, a session she thought had gone well, a client approaching grief, Zowie staying warm and steady throughout. The supervisor watched four minutes and paused the tape on Zowie's face. "What do you feel, right here, watching yourself?" Zowie said she looked calm. The supervisor agreed, and then gently pointed at the client on the screen, who had sighed, gone into her hands, and risen toward tears three separate times, and at Zowie, who at each rise had said something kind and general that landed like a soft blanket over a fire. "Your calm," the supervisor said, without cruelty, "is working very hard. Who taught you that feelings this size need blankets?"

Zowie drove home from that block certain she was done. Not because the supervisor was wrong, but because she was right, and being seen that accurately felt unsurvivable. The committee in her head had its best week in years. What kept her in was mundane: a scheduled phone call with a training peer, who confessed the same review had flattened him in block one, plus one honest hour in her own personal therapy, where she noticed that the wish to quit felt exactly like her clients' wish to cancel after their first real session. She had become, briefly, her own most instructive case.

She stayed. The blanket habit took a year of supervised repetitions to loosen, and it loosened. In her final block, watching her month-four tape again as an exercise, Zowie laughed out loud at the blankets, with something that was no longer shame. Mostly.

What this means for you: the training will find your defenses, because they run your clinical style, and meeting them on video is the tuition. Build supports before you need them: a peer, and ideally your own therapy. Everyone's month four is coming, and it is survivable by design.

12.4 What to Read Next

Here is the reading ladder, in order, with honest notes. Titles and authors only; full details live in the reference list at the back of this book.

After this book, go next to one of the two modern doorways. Jon Anders Lied's introduction is the new standard entry text, systematic and current, written for clinicians approaching the model fresh; its main barrier is price, as academic hardbacks and even the paperback run well beyond a trade book (Lied, 2025). Patricia Coughlin Della Selva's classic theory-and-technique volume is the time-tested alternative, denser but rich with case material (Coughlin Della Selva, 2004). It first appeared in 1996; the edition in print is the later reissue. Either works; pick by budget and tolerance for density.

Third, Jon Frederickson's big skills manual, the book working therapists keep on the desk: hundreds of concrete vignettes of what to actually say, organized by clinical problem (Frederickson, 2013). Fourth, Allan Abbass's advanced text on the spectrum of resistance and fragility, which will make Chapter 9.0 of this book look like the postcard version it is (Abbass, 2015). And fifth, when you want the deep water: the roadmap volume by ten Have-de Labije and Neborsky, and Davanloo's own selected papers, which are genuinely difficult and genuinely the source (Davanloo, 1990; ten Have-de Labije & Neborsky, 2012).

Two supplements earn their place at any rung: Malan and Coughlin Della Selva's book of transformed lives, the most readable case collection in the tradition, and, once training tempts you seriously, Rousmaniere on deliberate practice, which will reframe the video mortification as method (Rousmaniere, 2024).

You might be thinking that is a lot of books. It is five plus this one, spread over a year or two, and every one of them is cheaper than a single training day. Rung one is the best bargain in psychotherapy education.

12.5 Example

Not everyone's next step is a course, and Japji's ninety days are worth watching before you meet the plan in Appendix B.

Japji was a therapist in a rural area, two hundred miles from the nearest ISTDP trainer, with a training budget that year of approximately zero. What he had was this rung-one toolkit and some discipline, so he built a self-study season. Weeks one to four: he reread the two triangles until he could draw them cold, and began a practice journal, one entry per workday, recording a single observed moment, stimulus, feeling, anxiety sign, defense, from his own sessions. Nothing fancy; four lines a day.

Weeks five to eight: he added the body. One anxiety channel per fortnight, as Chapter 5.0 suggests, watched across his caseload, plus published demonstration videos in the evenings, sound off for the first pass, reading sighs and hands. He recruited a colleague into a fortnightly video call, and they drilled the sorting exercise from section 3.7 with fresh examples they wrote for each other, which turned out to be the single highest-value hour of the whole plan.

Weeks nine to twelve: he practiced the two safe skills from Chapter 8.0, the five-breath non-rescue and the once-per-session gentle noticing, and logged what happened. At day ninety he took stock, honestly. His questions had sharpened, three clients had gone visibly deeper, and his notes had a new column that his old notes lacked entirely: what the body did. He also logged the limits without flinching: twice he had spotted rising feeling and had no trained idea what to do next, and once he had backed off a foggy client correctly and known, precisely, that knowing-when-to-stop was the only ISTDP skill he actually possessed.

Japji's verdict, in his journal, deserves quoting because it is the right-sized ambition for rung one: "Ninety days did not make me an ISTDP therapist. It made me a therapist who sees more. Enrolling next year."

What this means for you: the distance between reading and training is not empty. There is a season of legitimate, structured, nearly free practice in it, and Appendix B hands you Japji's plan in checklist form.

12.6 When It Doesn't Work

The failure mode of training chapters is the permanent rung one. You finish the book inspired, bookmark two course pages, tell a colleague you are seriously considering core training, and then eleven days become eleven months, and the drafts folder wins. Zowie's committee is patient, and it holds seats for everyone: too junior, too senior, wrong profession, wrong country, and the chair reserved for they will see me work.

Why it happens: the next rung is the first one that involves being witnessed, and every instinct this book has described in clients, the avoidance of exposure, the management of feeling through delay, runs in therapists at full strength. You are not weak for stalling. You are a case study, which by now should feel almost companionable.

Three things to try. First, shrink the step below the step: not enrolling, not even emailing, just fifteen minutes on one trainer's website with the IEDTA directory open, today, vetting one name against the standards in section 12.1 (International Experiential Dynamic Therapy Association, n.d.). Second, convert the committee into an email: write to one training provider with your actual doubts, wrong profession, too long qualified, and let their answer, rather than your committee, rule on eligibility. Providers answer these questions weekly and kindly. Third, put a date on rung two only: one pre-core course, this year, as an experiment with an exit, which is all it is.

And if the honest answer after all that is not now, take it seriously and take the pressure off. Run Japji's ninety days instead, twice if you like. The ladder does not expire, and the clients you see more clearly in the meantime are not a consolation prize. They are the point.

12.7 The Road From Here

The ladder is standard worldwide: read and watch, then a pre-core course of workshop days for a few hundred dollars or pounds, then the three-year core training, small group, real caseload, supervised video, open to licensed professionals, then supervision as a way of life. The costs come in three currencies, money in the low thousands spread over years, time in steady background load, and pride, paid mostly at the video reviews, which turn out to be the fastest feedback loop in the business and the reason the training works.

Read Lied or Coughlin Della Selva next, then Frederickson, then Abbass, with Malan and Coughlin Della Selva's cases alongside. Vet any trainer against the IEDTA directory. And if the committee in your head is currently drafting reasons, remember it has a name in this model, and you know how it is worked with: seen kindly, honored for its history, and declined, today, in one fifteen-minute act.

One chapter of story remains, and it is short, and it is yours.

Conclusion: Walking Through the Door

Remember the note.

Back in the Introduction, before any triangles, this book asked you to write down two things: the name of one client who talks about feelings without ever seeming to feel them, and one question you hoped this model could answer. Go and find it if you can. Reading your own handwriting from the far side of twelve chapters is a small, private measurement of distance, and you have come farther than it felt like at the time.

Think about that client now. You can probably see things around them that were invisible when you wrote their name. Perhaps a favorite defense, with its history and its price. Perhaps which channel their anxiety takes when something true gets close. Perhaps the moment in your last session together when a feeling rose and something swept it politely off the table, and you, being then a person who had not read Chapter 3.0, let it go. The client has not changed. Your eyes have. That was this book's actual promise, made in the Introduction and now, hopefully, kept: not to make you an ISTDP therapist, but to move the model from rumor to understanding, and understanding changes what you see on Monday.

Morag, from the Introduction, would like her ending told. She sent the email she had been not-sending, sat through a pre-core course with her committee of doubts in full session, and discovered what Zowie discovered and what you may discover: that the people in ISTDP trainings are not intimidating experts but curious clinicians with the same twelve tabs open. She is in her first year of core training now. Her month four is coming, and she knows it is coming, which is more than most of us get. Some things in her practice changed early and stayed changed. She has never again, she says, accepted a weather report about a burning house.

And your question, the one on the note? Maybe it got answered somewhere in these pages. Maybe it sharpened into a better question, which is worth more. Either way, take it seriously as a compass. The curiosity that made you write it is the same force this model calls the healthy will, the part of a person that wants the true thing even when the true thing costs. Clients recover on the strength of it. Careers get rebuilt on it too.

So, one last time, the whole model on a note card. Buried feeling drives anxiety. Anxiety summons defense. Defenses cost, and the cost is called symptoms. Watch the body, honor the history, name the price, invite the feeling, and go only as fast as the system in front of you can bear. Everything else, the triangles, the channels, the pressure, the grading, the breakthroughs and their quiet consolidation, is that card, unfolded.

Here is your seven-day step, and then this book will stop assigning you things. Within the next week, do one of the following, sized to your season. Fifteen minutes with the IEDTA directory and one trainer's website. Or the first entry of Japji's practice journal, four lines about one moment in one session. Or order the next book on the ladder. One act, this week, while the reading is still warm in you.

The door is not locked. It never was. It just needed someone to show you the handle, and now you have seen it, and the rest is walking.

Thank you for reading, and good luck in the room.

Appendix A: Plain English Glossary

Anxiety pathways: The three channels through which anxiety discharges in the body. Striated muscle (tension and sighing, a green light), smooth muscle (gut and vascular symptoms, a slow-down signal), and cognitive-perceptual disruption (fog and unreality, a stop signal). See Chapter 5.0.

Breakthrough: The direct bodily experience of a previously buried feeling, as distinct from insight about it. Often accompanied by the surfacing of vivid memories. Also called unlocking. See Chapter 10.0.

Capacity: How much rising feeling a person's system can contain while keeping thinking and perception intact. Capacity is buildable. See Chapters 5.0 and 9.0.

Character defenses: Long-running defenses woven into personality itself, such as lifelong pleasing or permanent reasonableness. The load-bearing walls. See Chapter 6.0.

Cognitive-perceptual disruption: The third anxiety pathway. Thinking fogs, perception distorts, the room goes unreal. Always a stop signal. See Chapter 5.0.

Complex transference feelings: The mixture of irritation, fear, guilt, love, and buried old feeling that rises toward the therapist under sustained pressure. Its rise carries the past up with it. See Chapters 4.0 and 8.0.

Consolidation: The work after a breakthrough of connecting the felt experience to the pattern of a whole life, and testing new capacity in living relationships. Where change is actually secured. See Chapter 10.0.

Defense: Anything a person does, inside or outside awareness, to avoid experiencing a feeling. Every defense was a solution first. See Chapters 3.0 and 6.0.

Dynamic inquiry: Active, specific exploration of the presenting problem at the level of concrete moments rather than summaries. See Chapter 7.0.

Fragility: A precise term for limited capacity: anxiety that leaves the muscles early for the gut or the fog, and defenses that distort reality. Calls for the graded format. See Chapter 9.0.

Graded format: The adapted ISTDP for fragile clients. Raise feeling slightly, stop, regulate, observe the cycle together, repeat, building capacity across many gentle repetitions. See Chapter 9.0.

Head-on collision: An advanced, structured confrontation with the client's whole resistance at once, reserved for trained hands, high resistance, and an established alliance. See Chapter 8.0.

ISTDP: Intensive Short-Term Dynamic Psychotherapy. A therapy built on the claim that emotional avoidance drives symptoms and that directly experiencing avoided feeling, with a steady ally, produces deep change. See Chapter 1.0.

Pressure: Sustained invitation toward feeling, calibrated against the anxiety channels, inside an explicit alliance. Consistency, not volume. See Chapter 8.0.

Psychodiagnosis: The continuous reading of each client response against the triangle of conflict, including which anxiety channel is active and which defenses appear. Determines pacing and route. See Chapters 5.0 and 7.0.

Resistance: The defensive system operating against the therapy itself, protecting the person from the feelings the work approaches. Worked with, never fought. See Chapters 6.0 and 8.0.

Self-attack: A defense that reroutes feeling meant for someone else back onto its owner. Strongly tied to depression in this model. See Chapters 3.0 and 6.0.

Smooth muscle pathway: The second anxiety channel: gut, airways, and blood vessels. Stomach knots, nausea, migraine-type symptoms. A slow-down signal. See Chapter 5.0.

Striated muscle pathway: The first anxiety channel: voluntary muscles. Sighing, clenching, tension. Broadly a green light that feeling is rising within capacity. See Chapter 5.0.

Tactical defenses: Quick, in-the-moment avoidance moves such as subject changes, little laughs, and vagueness. The pawns of the system. See Chapter 6.0.

Transference: Responding to a present person with feelings and strategies built for a past one. Old learning generalizing. Treated in ISTDP as the work arriving, not a complication. See Chapter 4.0.

Trial therapy: Davanloo's name for the extended first encounter that is simultaneously genuine help and a live assessment of the system's response to rising feeling. See Chapter 7.0.

Triangle of conflict: Malan's map of the internal machinery: feeling at the bottom, anxiety and defense above, always in that causal order. Not the drama triangle. See Chapter 3.0.

Triangle of persons: Malan's map of where the machinery runs: past figures, current figures, and the therapist in the room. Linking its corners is an engine of brief therapy. See Chapter 4.0.

Unconscious therapeutic alliance: The deep cooperation that rises beneath the surface struggle: the client's healthy side actively joining the work, offering memories, dreams, and feeling. See Chapter 8.0.

Unlocking the unconscious: Davanloo's phrase for the breakthrough of buried feeling into direct experience, with the associated surfacing of memory. See Chapter 10.0.

Appendix B: The Ninety-Day Plan

Japji's twelve weeks, from section 12.5, in the form he actually used them. Nothing here requires training, a supervisor, or anyone's permission. Every activity is either something you do alone with your own notes, something you do with published material, or one of the two safe skills marked in Chapter 8.0. Nothing on this list authorizes you to use pressure, challenge, or any uncovering technique with a client.

Work it in order. The weeks build on each other, and the third block will not land if you skip the first.

Weeks One to Four: The Maps

Draw both triangles cold: On blank paper, from memory, until it is automatic. Feeling at the bottom, anxiety and defense above. Past figures, current figures, therapist. Test yourself on a Monday, not on the day you reread the chapter.

Start the journal: One entry per working day, four lines, no more. The stimulus. The feeling you think rose. The anxiety sign you saw. The defense that arrived. One moment from one session. If you noticed nothing that day, write that you noticed nothing, because that is also data.

Redo the sorting drill: Return to section 3.7 and work it again. Getting some wrong on a second pass is normal and is the entire point of a drill.

Say nothing yet: Weeks one to four are observation only. No naming, no interpreting, no experimenting on anyone.

Weeks Five to Eight: The Body

One channel per fortnight: Weeks five and six, watch only for sighs, clenching, jaw, and shoulders. Weeks seven and eight, watch only for the somatic complaints: the stomach, the nausea, the sudden exhaustion. Leave the third channel alone. You will recognize fog when it arrives, and the instruction never changes, which is to stop.

Videos with the sound off: Fifteen minutes of published demonstration footage in the evening. First pass silent, reading hands and breath only. Second pass with sound. The signal is far easier to see when the words are not competing for your attention.

Recruit one colleague: A fortnightly call. Write three fresh sorting items each for the other person, drawn from your own caseloads with the details changed. Japji rated this the highest-value hour of the whole plan, and he was right.

Keep the journal running: By week eight it should contain a column your old notes never had, which is what the body did.

Weeks Nine to Twelve: The Two Safe Skills

Practice not rescuing: When a client sits in productive discomfort, count five slow breaths before you speak. Log every time you managed it and every time you did not. The failures are more instructive.

One honest noticing per session: Once, gently, offered as an observation and not a verdict. I notice we moved away from your mother just as tears came. Once. Then let it go, whatever they do with it.

Keep watching the channels: This is the foundation the other two skills stand on, and it is the skill that keeps improving after the ninety days end.

Add nothing else: The temptation at week ten is to try something out of Chapter 8.0. That is precisely the temptation Chapter 8.0 warned you about, and it arrives on schedule.

Day Ninety: The Stock-Take

Sit down with the journal and answer four questions in writing. Writing, not thinking, because the difference is the whole exercise.

What do I see now: that I could not see in week one?

Which client, specifically: do I understand differently, and what changed in how I understand them?

Where did I run out of road: List every moment you spotted rising feeling and had no trained idea what to do next. Be honest and be specific. That list is the argument for training. It is not evidence against you.

What is my next step: sized to my actual season: a pre-core course, another ninety days, or nothing yet? All three are legitimate answers.

Japji's own verdict is worth borrowing as the right-sized ambition. Ninety days did not make him an ISTDP therapist. It made him a therapist who sees more.

What This Plan Does Not Do

It does not train you. It does not license you to use pressure, challenge, or the head-on collision. It does not qualify you to work with a fragile client any differently than you would have before you opened this book. What it does is convert reading into noticing, which is the only part of this model that transfers without a supervisor, and which is worth having whether or not you ever enroll in anything at all.

References

Abbass, A. (2015). *Reaching through resistance: Advanced psychotherapy techniques*. Seven Leaves Press.

Abbass, A., Kisely, S., & Kroenke, K. (2009). Short-term psychodynamic psychotherapy for somatic disorders: Systematic review and meta-analysis of clinical trials. *Psychotherapy and Psychosomatics, 78*(5), 265–274. https://doi.org/10.1159/000228247

Abbass, A. A., Kisely, S. R., Town, J. M., Leichsenring, F., Driessen, E., De Maat, S., Gerber, A., Dekker, J., Rabung, S., Rusalovska, S., & Crowe, E. (2014). Short-term psychodynamic psychotherapies for common mental disorders. *Cochrane Database of Systematic Reviews, 2014*(7), Article CD004687. https://doi.org/10.1002/14651858.CD004687.pub4

Abbass, A., Town, J., & Driessen, E. (2012). Intensive short-term dynamic psychotherapy: A systematic review and meta-analysis of outcome research. *Harvard Review of Psychiatry, 20*(2), 97–108. https://doi.org/10.3109/10673229.2012.677347

Anestis, M. D., Anestis, J. C., & Lilienfeld, S. O. (2011). When it comes to evaluating psychodynamic therapy, the devil is in the details. *American Psychologist, 66*(2), 149–151. https://doi.org/10.1037/a0021190

Barlow, D. H., Farchione, T. J., Sauer-Zavala, S., Latin, H. M., Ellard, K. K., Bullis, J. R., Bentley, K. H., Boettcher, H. T., & Cassiello-Robbins, C. (2017). *Unified protocol for transdiagnostic treatment of emotional disorders: Therapist guide* (2nd ed.). Oxford University Press.

Bowen, M. (1978). *Family therapy in clinical practice*. Jason Aronson.

Coughlin Della Selva, P. (2004). *Intensive short-term dynamic psychotherapy: Theory and technique*. Karnac Books. (Original work published 1996)

Davanloo, H. (1990). *Unlocking the unconscious: Selected papers of Habib Davanloo, MD*. Wiley.

Fosha, D. (2000). *The transforming power of affect: A model for accelerated change*. Basic Books.

Frederickson, J. (2012, November 27). *The triangle of conflict*. ISTDP Institute. https://istdpinstitute.com/2012/the-triangle-of-conflict/

Frederickson, J. (2013). *Co-creating change: Effective dynamic therapy techniques*. Seven Leaves Press.

Greenberg, L. S. (2015). *Emotion-focused therapy: Coaching clients to work through their feelings* (2nd ed.). American Psychological Association. https://doi.org/10.1037/14692-000

Hayes, S. C., Strosahl, K. D., & Wilson, K. G. (2011). *Acceptance and commitment therapy: The process and practice of mindful change* (2nd ed.). Guilford Press.

International Experiential Dynamic Therapy Association. (n.d.). *Home*. Retrieved July 24, 2026, from https://iedta.net

ISTDP UK. (n.d.). *Training courses*. Retrieved July 24, 2026, from https://www.istdp.org.uk/training/

Johansson, R., Town, J. M., & Abbass, A. (2014). Davanloo's intensive short-term dynamic psychotherapy in a tertiary psychotherapy service: Overall effectiveness and association between unlocking the unconscious and outcome. *PeerJ, 2*, Article e548. https://doi.org/10.7717/peerj.548

Karpman, S. B. (1968). Fairy tales and script drama analysis. *Transactional Analysis Bulletin, 7*(26), 39–43.

Lied, J. A. (2025). *An introduction to intensive short-term dynamic psychotherapy: Foundations of clinical practice*. Routledge.

Lilliengren, P., Johansson, R., Lindqvist, K., Mechler, J., & Andersson, G. (2016). Efficacy of experiential dynamic therapy for psychiatric conditions: A meta-analysis of randomized controlled trials. *Psychotherapy, 53*(1), 90–104. https://doi.org/10.1037/pst0000024

Lilliengren, P., Mechler, J., Lindqvist, K., Maroti, D., & Johansson, R. (2025). The efficacy of experiential dynamic therapies: A 10-year systematic review and meta-analysis update. *Clinical Psychology & Psychotherapy, 32*(3), Article e70086. https://doi.org/10.1002/cpp.70086

Malan, D. H. (1979). *Individual psychotherapy and the science of psychodynamics*. Butterworths.

Malan, D. H. (1980). The most important development in psychotherapy since the discovery of the unconscious. In H. Davanloo (Ed.), *Short-term dynamic psychotherapy* (pp. 13–23). Jason Aronson.

Malan, D., & Coughlin Della Selva, P. (2006). *Lives transformed: A revolutionary method of dynamic psychotherapy*. Karnac Books.

Rousmaniere, T. (2024). *Deliberate practice for psychotherapists: A guide to improving clinical effectiveness* (2nd ed.). Routledge.

Shedler, J. (2010). The efficacy of psychodynamic psychotherapy. *American Psychologist, 65*(2), 98–109. https://doi.org/10.1037/a0018378

ten Have-de Labije, J., & Neborsky, R. J. (2012). *Mastering intensive short-term dynamic psychotherapy: A roadmap to the unconscious*. Karnac Books.

Town, J. M., Abbass, A., Stride, C., & Bernier, D. (2017). A randomised controlled trial of intensive short-term dynamic psychotherapy for treatment resistant depression: The Halifax depression study. *Journal of Affective Disorders, 214*, 15–25. https://doi.org/10.1016/j.jad.2017.02.035

Town, J. M., Abbass, A., Stride, C., Nunes, A., Bernier, D., & Berrigan, P. (2020). Efficacy and cost-effectiveness of intensive short-term dynamic psychotherapy for treatment resistant depression: 18-month follow-up of the Halifax depression trial. *Journal of Affective Disorders, 273*, 194–202. https://doi.org/10.1016/j.jad.2020.04.035

www.ingramcontent.com/pod-product-compliance
Lightning Source LLC
LaVergne TN
LVHW022107200926
848481LV00003B/1092
9798905996870